Do You Call This a Life?

Gerbert van Loenen

Gerbert van Loenen

Do You Call This A Life?

Blurred Boundaries in the Netherlands' Right-to-Die Laws

RossLattner   London Canada

Library and Archives Canada Cataloguing in Publication

Loenen, Gerbert van, 1964-
[Hij had beter dood kunnen zijn. English]
Do you call this a life? : blurred boundaries in the Netherlands' right-to-die laws /
Gerbert van Loenen ; translation: Maggie Oattes; editor: Jim Ross.

UPDATED, REVISED TRANSLATION OF *Hij had beter dood kunnen zijn.*
Oordelen over andermans leven, AMSTERDAM, VAN GENNEP, 2009.
RESEARCH FOR THIS BOOK WAS SUPPORTED BY: *the Fonds Bijzondere*
Journalistieke Projecten (fondsbjp.nl).

Includes bibliographical references.
Issued in print and electronic formats.
Text in English; translated from the Dutch.
ISBN 978-1-897007-28-0 (pbk.).--ISBN 978-1-897007-29-7 (pdf)

1. Right to die--Law and legislation--Netherlands. I. Oattes, Maggie, transla-
tor II. Title. III. Title: Hij had beter dood kunnen zijn. English.

KKM3121.5.L6313 2015   344.49204'197   C2015-900152-8
                                                      C2015-900153-6

TRANSLATION: *Maggie Oattes*   EDITOR: *Jim Ross*
COVER DESIGN: *Jim Ross*
PUBLISHED BY: *Ross Lattner Educational Consultants*
147 William Street, London, Ontario, Canada N6B 3B4
519-639-0412
books@rosslattner.ca

Table of Contents

Table of Contents

Table of Contents

List of Abbreviations

BOSK   People With Physical Disabilities And Their Parents

CAL   Commission for Acceptability of Life Terminating Action

CDA   Christian Democratic Appeal

D66   Left-wing liberal political party *Democrats 66*

ICRC   UN International Convention on the Rights of the Child

JPV   Dutch Lawyers' Association Pro Vita

KNMG   Royal Dutch Medical Association

KVZ   Catholic Association of Care Institutions

LHV   Dutch Association of General Practitioners

NVAE   non-voluntary active euthanasia

NVIC   Netherlands Society of Intensive Care

NVK   Dutch Pediatric Association

NVVA   The Association of Geriatric Physicians

NVVE   Dutch Association for a Voluntary End to Life.

NVVE   *before 2005* Dutch Association for Voluntary Euthanasia

PPS   Public Prosecution Service

UMCG   Groningen University Hospital

VAE   voluntary active euthanasia

VVD   Right-wing libertarian party *People's Party for Democracy*

WBOPZ   Psychiatric Hospitals Compulsory Admission Act

Committee on Medical Ethics and Health Law of the Dutch Pediatric Association

Committee on Medical Ethics and Health Law

Central Committee Of Experts To Review Cases Of Active Termination Of Lives Of Newborns

Introduction

This is a view from within the Netherlands – the first country to enact right-to-die laws. Now that euthanasia and assisted suicide are being discussed across the Western world, it is worthwhile to take a look at the country that made the first moves in this direction.

This book challenges those who believe that it is easy to introduce right-to-die laws, and then restrict termination of life to just those people who want to die. In the Dutch example, what started as strictly 'euthanasia on request' also left room for non-voluntary euthanasia.

The Dutch were the first to regulate termination of life of severely handicapped or ill babies. Today, the debate in the Netherlands focuses on assisted suicide for elderly people who wish to die, but who are otherwise not dying. More importantly, what are the consequences of right-to-die laws for daily life? Do they undermine solidarity with people who are handicapped? Instead of being inviolable, life becomes just another option. Even the notion that we must help someone who becomes disabled becomes optional. These developments make the Netherlands a unique laboratory that the entire world should study.

Gerbert van Loenen is a Dutch journalist. From 2006 until 2014 he was deputy editor-in-chief of the Dutch daily newspaper *Trouw*. Prior to that, he was news correspondent in Germany for the same paper.

Van Loenen's committment to write this book arose from a deeply personal experrience. After his late partner suffered a severe brain injury, he was shocked by an acquaintance who said that his partner "would be better off dead." This is Gerbert van Loenen's analysis of the arguments that led to such a judgment.

*"This is the paradox of
the high-quality care in the Netherlands:
we have such lofty ideals about being human,
that we are dissatisfied
when a person does not meet those ideals,
despite our best care.*

*In this way
an idealistic image of humankind,
good care,
and a medical system that threatens people
can coexist together."*

Chapter 1

Self-Determination

The Ultimate Argument For Euthanasia

The Courageous Individual In Cinema

In the free West, the person we marry, where we live, what we do with our lives, are things we have the right to decide for ourselves. So why can't we decide how and when to die? Though few countries so far allow euthanasia, the issue is being debated in all Western countries. Nothing unusual about free debate. The Netherlands defines euthanasia as the intentional termination of another person's life at his own express request. On the face of it, this is in line with the notion that man can decide what to do with his own life. This chosen death may be looked upon sympathetically in all countries where self-determination is considered an important value.

And it shows – for example in the cinema. The individual who fights for his right to die with dignity works well as a screenplay, especially if he has to battle with the patronizing institutions that deny him this right. That such movies are made in the Netherlands, the country with the most far-reaching freedom to carry out euthanasia, will not come as a surprise. Yet in countries like Spain and the United States, where euthanasia is legally prohibited, successful movies have been released that are compatible with this image. The cinematic depiction of euthanasia as a form of self-determination by a free individual is spreading across the world. We will examine four examples from recent films.

MOVIE: *The Sea Within*

Consider the 2004 Spanish movie *The Sea Within*, [*Mare Adentro*] based on a true story. The protagonist, Ramon Sampedro, is the ultimate representation of the autonomous disabled individual: he is paralyzed from the neck down and in full possession of his faculties. Since his diving accident years ago Ramon, who can only move his head and speak, has been lying in bed. All things considered he is in high spirits. He is patiently cared for by his sister-in-law Manuela, but he wants to die – and this is not allowed under Spanish law.

Although Manuela takes care of him without any help from home care services or anyone else, she is not tired of him. She does not press him; she is completely unselfish, self-sacrificing and kind-hearted towards Ramon. The person in Ramon's circle who does exert pressure is a Roman Catholic priest, who is also a quadriplegic but who still wants to live. He calls on Ramon to do the same. This priest is portrayed in the movie as a bigot.

The storyline around Julia, Ramon's lawyer, is revealing. She is suffering from a progressive disease. She is still able to do more than Ramon, but her disease is getting worse. Julia says that she wants to help him die, and then end her own life. In the end, she shies away and lets him down. At the end of the movie, Ramon dies in an almost festive scene by cleverly evading the Spanish ban on euthanasia. At that point, we also see Julia again briefly. Her illness has clearly progressed – the disease has also affected her mind. We now see her in a wheelchair, staring out over the water. When she is told that Ramon is dead, it is clear she no longer has any idea who Ramon was.

So, brave Ramon chooses death, a death portrayed as an almost festive occasion. Julia on the other hand, balks at suicide and lives on, a life portrayed as sitting in a wheelchair, no memory, staring at the sea.

The Sea Within by director Alejandro Amenábar took the world by storm and was showered with awards.

MOVIE: *Million Dollar Baby*

This American film is similar. Perhaps the only difference is that the leading character does not become paralyzed until the end of the movie. Maggie Fitzgerald, a poor waitress, is the leading character. Purely by her will, she is transformed into a boxing champion. This comes to a cruel end at the height of her fame. During a fight against the German world champion, her neck is broken. Now on life support, completely helpless, she can only move her head. Her estranged family visits only in hopes of gaining possession of her hard-won assets. The only character loyal to Maggie is her manager. He eventually disconnects the respirator, and gives her a fatal injection.

This 2004 movie, directed by Clint Eastwood, won four Academy Awards, including best movie. It contains all of the elements of archetypal euthanasia: a person becomes completely paralyzed, is of sound mind and chooses death, aided by another courageous character.

MOVIE: *The Good Death*

Originally a play by Wannie de Wijn, it has been packing theatres since 2008. In the Netherlands, the heartland of euthanasia, the movie was released in 2012 under the name *De goede dood*. Ben is going to die of lung cancer. He has two brothers, one with a slight mental disability, the other one a successful businessman. After it has been explained to him, the mentally disabled brother sympathizes, and indicates that he believes that euthanasia really is the right choice for his sick brother Ben. The unsympathetic businessman-brother, on the other hand, asks a host of critical questions about the euthanasia directive of his brother, who is scheduled to die the next morning at 9 AM. Did his second wife put him up to it? What arrangements are made about the inheritance? Surely euthanasia is "not something Ben would want"? says the businessman-brother.

Hannah, the patient's wife, retorts that Ben does not understand "Because you're not sick." When Hannah does experience a moment of doubt, she asks the family doctor and friend: "This is what Ben really wants, isn't it?" The doctor answers Hannah without responding to the question: "You know, you are a brave person." Near the end, critically ill Ben says: "Now that God no longer exists, we have to do everything ourselves." Daughter: "Do you think that's better?" Ben: "At least it's less painful."

This play, produced with the assistance of Dutch euthanasia activists, Rob Jonquière and Eugène Sutorius, portrays euthanasia as a dignified, chosen death. Only the businessman-brother asks questions. The playwrights portray him as a coward who runs from death. The characters who support euthanasia, on the other hand, call each other courageous. Ben's final death scene is harmonious and warm.

MOVIE: *Simon*

Also from the Netherlands is the movie *Simon*, by Eddy Terstall. It is an ode to liberal, tolerant Amsterdam. The characters are homosexuals and soft-drug dealers, who co-exist in perfect harmony. When the leading character in this movie is diagnosed with a brain tumor, he opts for a "gentle, dignified" death, with the assistance of a physician. Simon's deathbed is portrayed as sunny and cordial, reminiscent of the death scene in *The Sea Within*.

Simon is an archetypal representation of euthanasia: a man, in full possession of his faculties, is struck by a serious illness and chooses euthanasia. He won't die in a hospital hooked up to machines, but at home, surrounded by the people he loves.

This 2004 movie won four Golden Calf awards, the most important movie award in the Netherlands.

Self-Determination Is Not All That Matters Here

The image of euthanasia in these films does not correspond to reality. In the first country to legalize euthanasia, the Netherlands, self-determination is not the key issue the filmmakers and their audience think it is. If you examine the developments in the Netherlands in detail, you have good reason to wonder whether things will be any different if euthanasia is legalized in other countries that are talking about it. The most important reason why there is no self-determination, no 'right to euthanasia', is that those who wish to die like this need a physician. Active termination of life requires a doctor who will administer the drugs in a lethal dose. In the case of assisted suicide the patient may be the one who takes the drugs, but he still needs a doctor to provide them.

The case law that has made euthanasia possible in the Netherlands focuses not on the patient, but on the physician and what he is allowed to do. The big fracture in the Dutch law took place in 1984, long before the law was changed. That year the Supreme Court of the Netherlands ruled that if a patient asks a physician for euthanasia, the physician can find himself in a 'situation of necessity' (the doctrine of *force majeure*: literally *stronger force* or *most compelling argument*). On the one hand the physician is duty-bound to save the patient's life. On the other hand he is obliged to relieve the patient's suffering. Responding to this conflict of interests, the High Court of the Netherlands found that the physician who performed euthanasia had not committed an offense.[1]

Throughout this time, public support for euthanasia had been growing in the Netherlands. This decision therefore drew much attention and was received with enthusiasm.

What the public failed to notice was that in 1984 the High Court explicitly rejected self-determination as grounds for accepting euthanasia. The central issue for the highest court was the patient's suffering, which placed the physician in a dilemma, a 'situation of necessity'. Many people who viewed euthanasia as a form of self-determination were so pleased with the High Court's ruling that they disregarded its arguments.

The 2001 Dutch Euthanasia Act that eventually resulted from the euthanasia debate also focused on physicians. Citizens were mentioned in the Euthanasia Act as persons who "may request" euthanasia, but clearly, they could not demand it. There was no 'right to euthanasia'. Earlier case

---

1   For this High Court decision see, for example, Tijdschrift voor Gezondheidsrecht, March/April 1985, pp. 90-100

law and the final 2001 Euthanasia Act both determined that there must be 'hopeless and unbearable suffering'. It is not up to the patient, it is the physician's job to determine whether there is such suffering.

The patient who wants to die autonomously, needs a doctor. This automatically restricts his autonomy. Unlike the patient, who dies, the physician has to answer for his actions afterwards. For this reason, the case law and the legislation both focus on the physician and the parameters of his freedom of action. Dutch euthanasia practice does not rest on the patient's self-determination – it rests on the doctor's pity. Self-determination is a far cry from pity. One could even say that pity is the opposite of self-determination. Pity, in essence, is patronizing. By substituting the word 'compassion', many writers hope to avoid the old-fashioned patronizing attitude conveyed by the word 'pity.'

Since the 1980s, debate and reality in the Netherlands have grown further apart. In movies, on television and on stage the key concept is invariably self-determination. When it becomes clear that barriers to euthanasia still exist, the public responds with incomprehension.

For those who are unable to express their will, such as people with mental disability or infants, self-determination simply does not apply. The general public understandably has less attention for these groups: the entire debate revolves around the autonomous, lucid citizen who decides in favor of euthanasia. Nevertheless, the most drastic and controversial developments taking place in the Netherlands are related to how legally incompetent persons are treated. This is the forgotten part, the dark side of euthanasia in the Netherlands.

The citizens of the Netherlands remain largely unaware of the debate that physicians, jurists and politicians initiated in the 1990's about termination of life without request. In the eighties the general public and the expert elite both focused on termination of life on request of the patient who wanted to decide his own fate. Since about 1990 the public debate has stagnated, left behind by the debate among the experts.

The public debate continues to focus mainly on euthanasia as termination at the request of persons who are capable of making that decision. The elite, in the meantime, is discussing a much more tangled question: can a physician decide for another person, who has no voice in the matter, that it is better for him to die? Cases involving newborns, people in a coma, people with multiple disabilities are more difficult to assess. The liberal arguments, based on self-determination by competent persons, are not very helpful here.

It has been quite a while since self-determination was the real issue for euthanasia in the Netherlands. For the past twenty years the public debate has been nothing more than a rerun of well-known arguments. It is out of step with the debates among elite professionals.

Unlike the public debate, this book is not limited to the autonomous characters of the movies. This book is also about persons in the Netherlands who are judged to be 'better off dead' – by others. This judgment has nothing to do with self-determination and everything to do with pity. Addressing the arguments that lead to the expression of such a judgment – "he'd be better off dead" – are the purpose of this book.

'Dying with dignity', as euthanasia supporters like to call it, is advocated in many countries besides the Netherlands. Belgium has taken the final step to euthanasia, and Luxembourg. The Canadian province of Quebec passed right-to-die legislation in 2014. Switzerland's position is slightly less extreme: one ordinary citizen can assist another to commit suicide. In Washington, Oregon and Vermont, physicians are allowed to assist their patients to commit suicide.

No one should ignore or conceal the Dutch example. Advocates of euthanasia must be challenged by the Netherlands' history. If champions of euthanasia think they can regulate 'dying with dignity' while avoiding the expansion in Dutch practice, then they must clearly formulate exactly what barriers they propose to erect to limit euthanasia to voluntary cases. This will only be possible if they expressly refer to the Dutch experience. Otherwise, they must expect a repetition of the Dutch developments.

There are no indications that this discussion is happening. All around the world we see exactly what initially happened in the Netherlands: the advocates of euthanasia refer to the classic examples of self-determination. A patient is seriously ill, is suffering and asks for termination of his life while fully conscious. That is exactly how the debate started in the Netherlands. Yet a debate in which advocates of euthanasia refer to the autonomy of man who should be allowed to decide his own life and death is valid only if termination of life is actually limited to people who did ask for it. This is not self-evident, as the Dutch example demonstrates. Perhaps the advocates of euthanasia in other countries actually do want to follow the Dutch example, including the cases in which the euthanized person is incapable of making the decision. If true, then let those advocates say so. However, they can no longer rely solely on the argument of self-determination, as they do now.

Chapter 2
Termination Of Life:

On Request If Possible,
Without If Necessary

The Dutch Euthanasia Act

"It is finished," said Els Borst[2] on Good Friday in 2001. The Dutch Minister of Public Health had just managed to get the Euthanasia Act passed by Parliament. What Dutch judges had developed by way of rules for euthanasia in case law since 1984, was now finally reflected in legislation. Some people reproached Borst for using these words that seem to be a quote of the words that, according to tradition, Jesus spoke just before dying on the cross on Good Friday. But Borst apologized to her critics "I did not know these words were spoken by Jesus."

The law that Borst managed to guide through the Dutch Parliament is considered the crown jewel of her party, the *Democrats 66*, established in the turbulent 1960s. This party boasts of being untainted by ideologies, and of wanting to clear the way for individual freedom. Thanks to this political achievement of Dutch liberalism, physicians are now allowed to assist their patients to die. The physician can terminate his patient's life either by administering a lethal dose of drugs, or by handing drugs to the patient to end his own life. The main conditions in law are (1) the physician has received a request from the patient who wants to die; (2)

---

2   On February 10, 2014, Els Borst was found dead. Dutch police concluded that she was a victim of either murder or manslaughter.

the physician is convinced that this patient is suffering hopelessly and unbearably, and (3) the physician has consulted a second physician.

In addition, the law requires the physician to report his actions to a review committee. The review committee determines whether he has observed these three conditions. If he has not, the law requires that they report the case to the Public Prosecution Service (PPS).

In 2013, the most recent year on which figures are available, the lives of 4,829 persons were terminated in accordance with the regulations of the Euthanasia Act. This is approximately 3.5 percent of all deaths in the Netherlands.[3] It is also a 15% increase over 2012.

Beyond the Euthanasia Act:
Termination Of Life Without Request

No sooner did the Dutch High Court accept euthanasia than physicians raised the next question. If any person with "hopeless and unbearable suffering" has the right to request euthanasia, is it not also allowed to help a legally incompetent person who suffers just as much? It is a perfectly logical question. After all, people who are not able to ask for euthanasia, like newborns for example, can also experience suffering.

There have been cases of euthanasia of a patient who does not ask for it. This happens between three hundred and one thousand times a year. In these cases the physician deliberately ends a patient's life without the patient's express request. Often it concerns persons who have not been able to request euthanasia because they are legally incompetent, for example newborns, or people in a coma. Termination of life *with* request is controversial; termination of life *without* request is even harder to justify. According to Dutch law, one of the legal conditions that must be met is that the patient must have asked the doctor to help him die. Termination of life is permitted only if requested by the patient.

And yet, the general public in the Netherlands does not get angry when cases of termination without request are revealed. In principle, Dutch law

---

3   Annual report 2013, Regional Euthanasia Review Committee

does not allow it, but judges have decided it is permissible. In these cases, the judge ruled the physician had acted in a 'situation of necessity'.

Any debate about this is limited to experts: physicians and jurists. The general public prefers to focus on the much simpler euthanasia discussion revolving around the self-determination of doomed and lucid individuals who say they want to die now.

Dutch politics has paid very little attention to termination of life without request. Despite the political division in the Netherlands, there is consensus on this point: none of the major political parties, left-wing, right-wing, traditional or populist, make an issue of termination of life without request.

We know that termination of life without request occurs in the Netherlands. Since 1991, there have been regular surveys among physicians about the decisions they make just before the death of their patients. Not just about euthanasia, this research is about all end-of-life medical decisions, ranging from discontinuing treatment and intensive palliative care to active 'termination of life'.[4] This is ingenious research, part of which consists of written questions to a sample of physicians who remain anonymous. They are asked to describe a recent death in their practice. The physicians are assured their answers cannot be traced back to them so they need not fear criminal prosecution. This survey has been repeated several times since then, and provides insight into the latest trends in end-of-life decisions.[5,6,]

Whether you are for or against the Dutch practice of 'termination of life' by physicians, there is no denying that efforts are being made to

4 P.J. van der Maas, J.M.M. van Delden and L. Pijnenborg, *Medische beslissingen rond het levenseinde*. Rapport van de Commissie onderzoek medische praktijk inzake euthanasie, Den Haag, SDU, 1991 [Medical end-of-life decisions. Report by the Committee to study the medical practice concerning euthanasia]

5 Maas, P.J. van der, J.J.M. van Delden, L. Pijnenborg, C.W.N. Looman, Euthanasia and other medical decisions concenring the end of life, Lancet 1991; 338: 669-704

6 Maas, P.J. van der, G. van der Wal, I. Haverkate e.a., Euthanasia and other end-of-life decisions in the Netherlands 1990-1995, N Engl J Med 1996; 335: 1699-1705

unearth the facts.[7,8,9,10] You may regard these figures as illustrations of the tradition of Dutch openness, of making any issue a subject of discussion. We have some idea what is taking place in the Netherlands. There is no similar research in other countries. This makes the Netherlands a unique laboratory for all the world to observe.

The Dutch figures

The first study, (van der Maas et. al, 1991), immediately revealed that termination of life without request was taking place in the Netherlands. In an estimated one thousand cases per year, or 0.8 percent of all deaths in the Netherlands, a physician provided a drug for the express purpose of ending a patient's life, without the patient actually asking for it. The term "express" is important in this definition: if a physician only provided the medication to alleviate pain, and he knew that expedited death was a potential side-effect, he was not considered to "expressly" hasten the end of life. The 0.8 percent referred only to those cases in which the physician administered drugs for the express purpose of ending the patient's life. The estimate of one thousand cases annually in the whole of the Netherlands was based on this sample.

In most of these one thousand cases of deliberate termination of life without request, the patients were not competent and therefore in no position to request anything. However, in fourteen percent of the cases of euthanasia without request, the patients whose lives were terminated by administering lethal drugs actually were competent. The physician decided, without asking them for their opinion, that it was better for

7   Wal, G. van der, P.J. van der Maas, J.M. Bosma, e. a., Evaluation of the notification procedure for physician-assisted death in the Netherlands, N Engl J med 1996; 335: 1706-1711

8   Onwuteaka-Philipsen B.D., A. van der Heide, D. Koper e.a., Euthanasia and other end-of-life decisions in the Netherlands in 1990, 1995, and 2001, Lancet 2003; 362: 395-399

9   Heide A. van der, B. D. Onwuteaka-Philipsen, M.L. Rurup et al., End-of-life practices in the Netherlands under the Euthanasia Act, N Engl J Med 2007; 356: 1957-1965

10   -Onwuteaka-Philipsen B., A. Brinkman-Stoppelenburg, C. Penning, G.J.F. de Jong-Krul, J.J.M. van Delden, A. van der Heide, Trends in end-of-life practices before and after the enactment of the euthanasia law in the Netherlands from 1990 to 2010: a repeated cross-sectional review, Lancet 2012, published online July 11, 2012

them that he ended their life.[11] The reasons the doctors gave for not consulting these competent patients, even though they were capable, were: "consultation would have done more harm than good" or "this course of action was clearly the best one for this patient."

Foreign observers reacted vehemently to these figures about unrequested termination of life. John Keown, an Englishman who had been monitoring the Dutch situation for years, wrote: "The hard evidence of the survey indicated that within six years of the promulgation of the guidelines for VAE (voluntary active euthanasia), NVAE (non-voluntary active euthanasia) was not uncommon. This is partly because of the inability of the vague and loose guidelines for VAE to ensure compliance. It is also partly because the underlying justification for VAE in the Netherlands appears not to be self-determination of the patient, but the principle that it is right to end the lives of certain patients because they are not worth living."[12]

Birgit Reuter, a German researcher, also reacted to the figures on unrequested 'termination of life.' She stressed that "this was to be expected." The justification of euthanasia in the Netherlands was not the self-determination of the patient, but the 'situation of necessity' of the physician who felt he should avoid suffering. This automatically reduced the importance of any request, or the absence of a request. The physician and his pity (compassion) occupied center stage. "This is the course the highest Dutch court took by deciding that a physician killing out of compassion could be justified due to *force majeure*. The assumption of a 'situation of necessity' for the physician already implied the acceptance of non-voluntary euthanasia. The request or consent of the person being killed is totally irrelevant to the question whether the physician acted in a situation of necessity."[13]

Whereas John Keown was criticized by Dutch experts (mostly in footnotes), Birgit Reuter has been completely ignored in the Netherlands.

---

11   van der Maas et al., 1991, p. 45-47

12   John Keown, *Euthanasia, Ethics and Public Policy. An Argument Against Legalisation*, Cambridge University Press, 2002, p. 123

13   Birgit Reuter, *Die gesetzliche Regelung der aktiven ärztlichen Sterbehilfe des Königreichs der Niederlande – ein Modell für die Bundesrepublik Deutschland?* Frankfurt, Peter Lang, 2000, p.235

This is so strange: whenever it has become clear that 'termination of life' without request actually happens, the Dutch reaction has been minimal. Although the public debate constantly repeated that lives are terminated only voluntarily, at the express request of the patient, these figures about unrequested termination of life barely received a response.

No wonder. Both the researchers and the committee that commissioned the 1991study started justifying the potentially shocking results immediately after publication. The committee members, including Supreme Court Attorney General professor J. Remmelink and the future Minister of Public Health Els Borst, wrote in their report: "The committee first of all observes that in those cases where no request is made for termination of life the active intervention of the physician is often unavoidable due to the patient's state of agony. For this reason the committee has labeled the life-terminating actions of the physician in these situations as assisted dying."[14]

The term they used, 'assisted dying', has no legal status in the Netherlands. Nevertheless, the committee used the term to exonerate physicians who ended the lives of people without their request. 'Assisted dying' was described by the committee as 'termination of life at the moment that vital organs begin to fail irreversibly'. The committee asserted that such termination of life should be considered part of normal medical practice. Indeed, they argued that in those cases euthanasia without request was simply "inescapable."

Further reasoning used by the committee is revealing: "The absence of a request for termination of life in these circumstances only complicates the decision making as compared to a situation in which there is a sustained, voluntary and carefully considered request for euthanasia. The ultimate justifying condition for the intervention in both types of situations is the unacceptably severe suffering." Paraphrasing the difficult prose of the Remmelink committee: pity or compassion is the reason that physicians sometimes end the lives of their patients. It is easier when the persons who are about to be killed for their own good consent to the

---

[14]   Op. cit., p.32.

termination, but it's not absolutely necessary. In other words, pity – not self-determination – is the essence of the Dutch practice of euthanasia.

Since the 1991 survey of the end-of-life decisions by physicians, the study has been repeated in 2001 and again in 2010. Whereas in the 2001 survey there were 950 cases of termination of life without request, according to the 2010 study termination of life without an express request by the patient occurred in an estimated 300 cases, i.e. in 0.2 percent of all deaths in that year.[15]

What is clear is that the attitude of physicians towards unrequested termination of life has become more restrained over the years. "In 1990 it was observed for the first time that not all cases of termination of life by a physician take place at the express request of the patient. One fourth of all physicians in the Netherlands at the time indicated having at one time or another acted in a life-terminating manner without being requested to, and another third indicated considering such action conceivable. In 1995 and 2001 these percentages had clearly dropped. In 2005, according to the physician survey, only 6 percent of all physicians indicated having performed life-terminating actions without express request and 7 percent indicated it was conceivable."[16] This is a considerable decrease, and it gives the impression that physicians are seriously reconsidering the medical practice that prevailed in the 1990s.

What About The Law?

From a medical perspective, according to the Remmelink committee that commissioned this study in 1990, there is "little difference" between termination of life with or without request, "as in both situations the patients are suffering severely."[17] Of course this is correct, but the perspective is indeed a purely medical one. It indicates that, in the eyes of the physicians, euthanasia is mainly a matter of pity toward their patient.

---

15   Heide, A. van der Heide, Brinkman-Stoppelenburg, A., Delden, H. van, Onwuteaka-Philipsen, B. Euthanasie en andere medische beslissingen rond het levenseinde. Sterfgevallenonderzoek 2010, Den Haag, ZonMW, 2012

16   Ibid., p. 111

17   Van der Maas *et al.*, op. cit., p. 32

From a legal standpoint one would expect the fact whether or not the patient made a request to die to make a difference. When euthanasia was on the rise one frequently heard the reassuring claim that self-determination was mandatory. Any person who 'terminated a life' without request would be guilty of murder. So how did the Dutch legislature, the Public Prosecution Service and the courts react to these cases of termination of life without request? Did they indeed view them as murder?

On the contrary. On the whole, the government, the parliament, the Public Prosecution Service (PPS) and the judges in the Netherlands sat back and waited. They left the initiative to the physicians and have generally followed what the physicians think, write and do. In the courtroom and in parliament the physicians had the initiative and in medical committees they tried to establish boundaries of permissible medical action. This was what happened in the case of euthanasia: the judiciary, and eventually the legislature, looked at the medical practice and subsequently followed along with it. This is what is happening now with respect to termination of the lives of people who do not request it.

Most people would expect the legislature and the courts to determine the boundaries for decisions about ending a person's life. But why would you need government, members of parliament, judges and public prosecutors to act, if they are not involved in setting and enforcing rules and regulations regarding termination of life? Isn't it odd that in a thoroughly regulated country like the Netherlands the government issues regulations about where to park your bicycles, smoking in bars and cutting down trees in backyards, but not for the deliberate termination of life by physicians?

It is interesting, especially for countries that are considering following the Dutch example, to analyze the developments that led to this situation. It is important to remember that these are all complicated cases, in which people are unmistakably suffering. Once the principle is accepted that termination of life is allowed to avoid severe suffering in some cases, determining a new boundary in everyday practice turns out to be difficult. The "personal request by the person who will die" proves to be a totally untenable boundary.

Most of the cases in which a physician opts for termination of life without request are never brought before a judge. When a physician does end a patient's life without request, and then reports it (which is not always done), the Public Prosecution Service often dismisses the case. PPS does not prosecute, for example, if other cases are considered more important. In February 1992, for example, the Attorneys General decided to back a colleague who had decided not to prosecute a physician who ended the life of a coma patient. The Minister of Justice concurred.[18] In November 1992 the Attorneys General also decided not to prosecute another physician who killed a coma patient, because the termination "was in fact tantamount to discontinuing a medically pointless treatment."[19]

When the PPS does prosecute a case of involuntary termination of life, they leave the decision to the judges. The judges rarely convict. Finding a physician guilty of 'termination of life without request' means the judge must actually call him a murderer, a term so harsh that judges tend to shy away from it. John Grifftiths, professor of Sociology of Law at the University of Groningen, has pointed out the mild sentences and semi-apologies that Dutch judges express to the few physicians who are convicted for decisions they made regarding the end of their patient's life. Griffiths concluded that criminal law is too blunt a weapon to monitor physicians who decide the end of other people's lives.[20] In the practice of termination of life without request, the role of the judiciary turns out to be minor.

---

18   John Griffiths, Heleen Weyers, Maurice Adams, *Euthanasia and Law in Europe*, Oxford and Portland, Oregon, Hart Publishing, 2008, p. 255

19   Keown, p. 118

20   John Griffiths et al., *Euthanasia and Law in the Netherlands*, Amsterdam, Amsterdam University Press, p. 273

Chapter 3
Termination Of Life In Babies

The Physician As His Own Legislator

So – if criminal law is too blunt an instrument, who monitors the physicians? Who decides how far a physician can go? In the Netherlands the people in charge of monitoring their actions are actually the physicians themselves. They determine the boundaries of their own actions.

Dutch law prohibits 'termination of life without explicit request'. Nevertheless, it happens. Physicians who actively ended lives without request have been acquitted in several essential court cases. One example, concerning newborn infants, demonstrates the development of this practice in the Netherlands in detail. Are physicians permitted to end the life of seriously ill or disabled newborns to avoid suffering?

In 2005 there was a revolution in this respect in the Netherlands. Requirements of due care had been formulated for physicians who deliberately ended the life of a newborn. In addition, the government had established a committee to review whether these due care requirements had been met in cases of termination of newborns' lives. Once you have these two things – rules, and a government-appointed committee to check that the rules are being observed – then you have taken two big steps on the road to accepting active termination of life in severely disabled or ill infants.

Who formulated these rules? Whose idea was it to create this committee? How did this breakthrough revolution come about? Why did the Netherlands take the lead in termination of life in severely ill or disabled infants? And why is it that, as was the case with euthanasia for many years, the law prohibited child euthanasia in general, but nevertheless allowed it in practice in certain circumstances?

It may come as a surprise that the people who in 2005 established the *Central Committee Of Experts To Review Cases Of Active Termination Of Lives Of Newborns* were two Christian-democratic politicians. The widespread notion that Christians and Christian politicians are generally pro-life and against euthanasia is untenable in the Netherlands. Here they seem to have played an essential role in enabling termination of life. Clemence Ross-van Dorp, Dutch State Secretary of Health, Welfare and Sport and Piet Hein Donner, Minister of Justice, both members of the *Christian Democratic Appeal* (CDA), informed the Second Chamber on November 29 2005 that such a committee was in the making. It would consist of a chair, an ethicist and three physicians tasked with reviewing cases in which physicians reported the termination of life of newborns and infants, in particular whether the physician had acted with 'due care'. The *Central Committee of Experts* would then prepare a joint expert opinion on this question, and present it to the Public Prosecution Service (PPS).

When Donner and Ross-van Dorp announced the formation of this committee, their opening statement was that termination of life without request was not permitted and was liable to punishment. This appears to be plain language, but those who think that ends the matter are mistaken. Sometimes, Donner and Ross-van Dorp argued, a physician will face a 'situation of necessity.' If a small patient is suffering severely, the physician wants to end the suffering; at the same time, he is also bound to respect life. Situations like these, Donner and Ross-van Dorp argued, may sometimes be considered 'situations of necessity' In that case, the physician is allowed to do what the law normally does not allow: to end the young life.

Donner and Ross-van Dorp cited two court decisions from the 1990s which showed that physicians who act with due care are indeed allowed to end the life of a newborn that suffers hopelessly and unbearably. The politicians adopted the requirements of 'due care' that had been developed in this case law.

In summary, the 2005 letter of Donner and Ross-van Dorp about termination of life in newborns says: the legislation doesn't permit termination of the lives of newborns, but if a physician meets the court's strict 'due care' requirements, the courts will permit it. We don't have to apply the criteria of due care too rigidly they wrote: "Not every violation of the rules of due care will necessarily lead to prosecution."

In their letter introducing the *Central Committee of Experts*, Donner and Ross-van Dorp employed reassuring words about ending newborn life: "Life is worthy of protection. This also applies to the disabled." This contradicts the rules described in the same letter for terminating the lives of seriously ill or disabled infants, but the authors do not elaborate on this paradox. The PPS was always free to deviate from the advice of the committee. Even if the committee concluded that a physician observed all criteria of due care, the PPS could still prosecute the physician. In this way, they reassured the public, monitoring remained possible.

The reassuring words of the minister and state secretary did not convince everyone. The Dutch patient organization for people with physical disabilities and their parents, BOSK, sent an outraged letter to the Dutch Second Chamber on December 8 2005. The organization stated that it had asked the state secretary for a system that would strengthen the rights of severely disabled children and the position of their parents. That did not happen. According to BOSK, the "hopeless and unbearable suffering" that Ross-van Dorp and Donner said must be present to justify euthanasia is a subjective concept. "BOSK has heard a great many testimonials about the quality of life from people directly involved that are often diametrically opposed to the statements and prognoses of medical professionals." When the committee announced that violations of the requirements of 'due care' would not always result in criminal prosecution, BOSK was not reassured.

So why did Donner and Ross-van Dorp write this introductory letter in the first place? Their letter mentioned legal rules, and the formation of a committee to enforce those rules. Did they in fact accept certain circumstances under which newborns in the Netherlands can be euthanized? The reason is that when Donner and Ross-van Dorp wrote their letter, they were responding to a written request, dated January 29 2003, from the *Royal Dutch Medical Association* KNMG, the *Dutch Pediatric Association* NVK, and the Dutch right-to-die association NVVE, urging the government to arrange a review and reporting procedure for termination of life without request.

The organizations KNMG, NVK and NVVE made this request because for many years there had been cases of termination of life of newborns without the Public Prosecution Service hearing about it. The cases that did get reported to the PPS were not prosecuted. In short: the lives of newborns were already being terminated, but there was no review. From their perspective, the implementation of the central expert committee was a measure that would increase control of euthanasia of newborns.

Moreover, by that time the courts had ruled in two cases that termination of life of newborns was permissible. In two landmark cases – the *Prins* case (1995) and the *Kadijk* case (1996) – the court rulings allowed termination of life of newborns, if they are likely to die in the near future and will suffer severely until then. Both cases applied the doctrine of *force majeure*: a physician may decide that the prevention of suffering has priority over preservation of life. Since then, the PPS has stopped prosecuting similar cases of termination of life in newborns.[21]

The *Prins* case concerns Dr. Prins, who in March 1993 delivered a baby with spina bifida, hydrocephalus, deformed hands and feet, and the lower part of her body paralyzed. According to the physicians her crying indicated that she was in pain. They decided to forego medical treatment. The life expectancy of the child was limited to a few months. Because of the child's pain, gynecologist Prins ended her life after three days at the request of her parents.

The Minister of Justice Donner urged the PPS to prosecute this case,

---

21   Alex Bood, Levensbeëindiging bij pasgeborenen. De uitdaging voor de centrale deskundigencommissie, *Nederlands Juristenblad*, 2007, 36 [Termination of life in newborns. The challenge for the central expert committee]

not so much to punish Prins, but rather for the development of case law. On appeal, Prins was acquitted by the court on the grounds of the doctrine of *force majeure*. The doctors had already decided not to treat the infant, who was expected to die soon. In the meantime the pain required treatment. Experts who were consulted told the court that pain relief was possible, but had disadvantages. One expert said that, as all treatment options had been exhausted, pain relief would have been 'medically pointless'. The court adopted the latter advice and concluded that "medical treatment in the form of pain relief was medically futile." The judges reasoned that Prins, by choosing termination of life, "has acted in accordance with scientifically sound medical understanding and in accordance with current medical ethical standards."[22]

One year later a similar case against Dr. Kadijk was brought before the court. A baby was born with Trisomy-13, a very serious chromosome disorder which results in death in the first year of life in 90 percent of all cases. The baby girl had a cleft lip and palate, two skin and skull defects, a pointed forehead, poor kidney function, deformed hands and fingers, low-set ears, upward slanting eyes. Furthermore, she went into cardiac arrest soon after birth and had trouble breathing. Doctor Kadijk and the baby's parents decided not to treat the child, and to bring her home. However, at home the cerebral membrane bulged out of the girl's skull, resulting in pain. After consultation, Kadijk decided to terminate her life.

Again, Minister of Justice Donner urged the PPS to prosecute Dr. Kadijk for the sake of developing case law. Again, the court decided on appeal that Kadijk could claim the defence of *force majeure*.

This time, the court based its decision on two earlier reports by physicians, and quoted them extensively. "The report *To Act Or Not? Boundaries Of Medical Practice In Neonatology* [*doen of laten? Grenzen van het medische handelen in de neonatologie*] by the *Dutch Pediatric Association* NVK describes that "consensus cannot be reached about deliberate termination of life in a situation in which after careful

---

22   De zaak-Prins, Hof Amsterdam November 7 1995, *TvGR* 1996, p. 30-36 [The Prins case]

consideration medical treatment of a newborn is discontinued primarily for reasons of limited future quality of life, and the newborn does not die in the immediate future, but that almost all physicians respect the opinions of those who choose this option, even if they themselves would be unable to justify it."

The second report quoted by the court in Kadijk's defence was produced by the KNMG's own Commission for the Acceptability of Life Terminating Action. The court quoted the medical commission: "If a situation develops of unnecessary extension and/or exacerbation of suffering, then it is the opinion of the commission that it can indeed be morally acceptable to proceed with the administration of euthanasia drugs." The court found that Kadijk acted in accordance with the prevailing medical ethical standards as described in the reports.[23]

It is remarkable that the court should come to this solid conclusion, considering that the doctors' opinions in those medical reports were divided. Opponents of euthanasia, who are definitely to be found among Dutch physicians, did not voice their opposition loudly and clearly. On the contrary, they felt they had to respect the opinions of their colleagues who did consider termination of life without request an option. The court then concluded that the medical profession in general apparently considered euthanasia without request permissible under specific circumstances. In this way, a fraction of the physicians in the Netherlands managed to accomplish a radical change – they made possible the termination of life without request.

These two cases opened the door to termination of life without request in newborns. The same argumentation that convinced the Supreme Court to allow euthanasia in the Netherlands was used here: a physician may find himself in a situation of necessity when his patient is suffering severely and the physician can do little about it except end the patient's life. Again we see the far-reaching implications of the 1984 decision of the Supreme Court, when "*force majeure* in the sense of a situation of necessity" made its entry into the Dutch euthanasia debate.

---

23   De zaak-Kadijk, Hof Leeuwarden April 4 1996, *TvGR* 1996, p. 284-291 [The *Kadijk* case]

This concept has been used, first to untie the legal ban on termination of life on request, and now also on termination of life without request. "*Force majeure* in the sense of necessity" used as an escape route: acts that are generally prohibited by law can be allowed in certain circumstances. Under *force majeure*, euthanasia was effectively legal for many years before the Dutch law had been amended. And now, following the same path, termination of life in newborns under strict conditions is becoming legal, although the law still does not allow it.

When they decided in the 1990s that the physician of an incompetent patient can find himself in a 'situation of necessity' that made termination of life an acceptable option, the courts based their decisions on what physicians themselves deemed acceptable. Especially in the *Kadijk* case the court extensively quoted two reports drawn up by physicians to determine boundaries: *To Act or Not?* and the *Report By The Commission For The Acceptability Of Life Terminating Action.*

The government took these cases as the starting point for setting up the *Central Committee of Experts* to review termination of life in newborns. They instructed the expert committee, perhaps unnecessarily, to pay special attention to what physicians had already discussed.

In short, two medical commissions wrote recommendations on whether it is acceptable to end the life of newborns. Twice the courts concluded that physicians who have terminated the life of disabled infants should not be prosecuted because they acted in accordance with accepted medical standards on these recommendations. The Public Prosecution Service subsequently used the court decisions as the basis for its policy to not prosecute similar cases in future. And this, finally, is the basis for the government's assumption that termination of life in newborns is sometimes allowed in accepted medical practice.

In the case of termination of life in newborns, the government and the judiciary follow the physicians. If the physicians are divided, they follow the physicians with the most radical opinions.

A Next Step: The Groningen Protocol

The boundaries of termination of life have not yet been established in the Netherlands, so the debate among physicians continues. Ten years ago, several influential pediatricians proposed going one step further. They proposed to include newborns who suffer seriously illness or disabilities, but who could survive without intensive medical care. Is it acceptable to end their lives because their illness or disabilities cause them severe suffering?

By 2005, this more radical form of life termination of newborns became regulated in the Groningen Protocol, a set of guidelines drawn up by the Academic Hospital Groningen, now renamed Groningen University Medical Center.[24] The Groningen Protocol has caused a stir in the Netherlands and abroad.

The 'due care' requirements in the Groningen Protocol are not obviously spectacular to anyone familiar with the earlier Dutch euthanasia discussion. The protocol entails a few procedural requirements: the physician who terminates the life of an infant must consult an independent colleague, the parents must consent, the termination of life must take place in a careful manner and the physician must declare that the child in question suffers hopelessly and unbearably.

New was the category of people to whom the Groningen protocol applies: seriously ill or disabled newborns who could survive on their own and were therefore not dependent on intensive medical treatment. Whereas the earlier *Prins* and *Kadijk* cases concerned euthanasia of infants whose treatment options were exhausted but would not die immediately, under the Groningen Protocol the seriously ill or disabled infants in question were able to survive. Their survival, however, would be deemed undesirable because their illness or disability would cause severe suffering.

---

24   See E. Verhagen and P.J.J. Sauer, The Groningen Protocol – euthanasia in severely ill newborns, *New England Journal of Medicine*, 2005, p. 959-962; and A.A.E. Verhagen, *End-of-life decisions in Dutch neonatal intensive care units*, diss. Rijksuniversiteit Groningen, 2009, Zutphen, Paris Legal Publishers, 2008, p. 26

Many critics, both within and outside the Netherlands, apparently do not understand this distinction. They think that the Groningen Protocol regulates termination of life in newborn infants in general, and this worries them. In reality, by the time the Groningen Protocol was introduced the courts in the Netherlands had already ruled on two occasions that termination of the lives of infants is acceptable, if the physician's goal is to avoid the suffering of infants for whom the doctors can do nothing. In reality, the Groningen protocol regulates life termination in babies with a longer life expectancy.[25]

We might question whether foreign critics of the Groningen Protocol would be reassured if they understood this nuance. Foreign critics of the Groningen Protocol do not realize that the situation in the Netherlands has already developed further than they know.

The *Dutch Pediatric Association* NVK views the 2005 Groningen Protocol as a national guideline. The physicians who formulated the Protocol were assisted by the Public Prosecution Service, who informed the physicians on the legal limits and opportunities provided by the earlier court decisions. Had the PPS intended to prosecute these actions, it obviously would not have provided this assistance. Their objective was clearly to develop new rules and establish a new boundary.

In summary: through the *Prins* and *Kadijk* cases, termination of life in ill and disabled infants became acceptable in practice if the physician declared that the infant suffered hopelessly and unbearably. Initially this was to apply only to the infants for whom it had already been decided that further medical treatment was pointless, resulting in a painful situation of necessity. Once the courts accepted this form of life termination, the PPS stopped prosecuting similar cases.

---

25   Eduard Verhagen, co-author of the Groningen Protocol uses a different definition and emphasizes that what is regulated in the protocol is in line with what the courts have already accepted. In his opinion the protocol applies to children that survive outside a NICU and suffer hopelessly and unbearably. Because the Prins and Kadijk cases also involved children that survived outside the NICU and suffered hopelessly and unbearably, he views the protocol as a logical consequence of those cases. (interview March 16 2009).

The 2005 Groningen Protocol endorsed termination of life for disabled infants for whom no decision has been made to forego life-prolonging medical treatment and who could survive on their own. Legislation to permit ending the life of a disabled infant who does not need intensive medical care has not yet been decided. The fact that physicians have already regulated this in their own Groningen Protocol, realized with the help of the PPS and unopposed by government officials, suggests that this form of life termination also has a good chance of being accepted in the Netherlands.

This new, liberalized boundary was not determined by the Dutch legislators in a public assembly in parliament. The physicians themselves, in committee meetings, in reports, and in a hospital in Groningen, have attempted to set the boundaries of what is acceptable and what is not. They, or at least the high-profile pediatricians who support the option of active life termination, are responsible for this radical change. The courts, and subsequently the PPS and the government, simply followed these physicians.

Euthanasia Expands to Prevent Future Suffering

The discussion within the physicians' committees in the Netherlands continued. The next question: can the life of an infant who is not suffering at this moment, but might suffer in the future, be terminated to avoid this future suffering? In June 2007, the *Committee on Medical Ethics and Health Law of the Dutch Pediatric Association* proposed to make this possible. "It seems unreasonable that physician and parents must always postpone their decision until the unbearable suffering has started."[26]

What future suffering did physicians want to avoid by ending the infant's life today? As it turns out, they were worried about three issues: the baby's expected inability to communicate, the impact of the treatment

---

26 A.A.E. Verhagen, M.A.H.B.M. van der Hoeven, J.B. van Goudoever, M.C. de Vries, A.Y.N. Schouten-van Meeteren en M.J.I.J. Albers, *Uitzichtloos en ondraaglijk lijden en actieve levensbeëindiging bij pasgeborenen, Nederlands Tijdschrift voor Geneeskunde,* 2007; 151: 1474-1477 [*Hopeless and unbearable suffering and active termination of life in newborns*]

on the baby, and the anticipated life expectancy of the newborn.

The latter criterion requires some explanation: the pediatricians felt that the higher the life expectancy of a disabled infant, the stronger the reason to opt for life termination now, because the future suffering might drag on for so long.

The Dutch Health Council followed a similar path. In 2007 they pointed out that a physician should not only relieve distress, he must also prevent it. It does not make sense to wait until the suffering actually occurs; the life of the infant should be ended before this happens, according to the *Health Council Committee on Health Ethics and Health Law*.[27]

However, a new boundary appeared to be materializing on this frontline of the Dutch euthanasia debate. The government-appointed commission that reviewed cases of euthanasia in infants rejected terminating the life of infants for reasons of future suffering. Active euthanasia could only be an option if the infant was suffering right now.

In its annual report, the committee described the difficult discussion with the physicians on this issue.[28] "According to the physicians, the requirement of actual unbearable suffering is in many cases difficult to apply to newborns with very severe defects ...doctors and parents can agree that it is better for these children not to live because of the anticipated very poor quality of life." Under the current regulations, the physicians realized, euthanasia was not allowed if the infants were not suffering at that time. Should those regulations be relaxed? No, said the committee explicitly: "The committee finds that active euthanasia of newborns is unacceptable if there is no situation of suffering. If the child does not suffer, there can be no decision to end its life."

---

27   Alex Bood, Levensbeëindiging bij pasgeborenen. *De uitdaging voor de centrale deskundigencommissie, NJB*, 2007/36 [*Termination of life in newborns. The challenge for the central expert committee*]

28   Gecombineerd Jaarverslag van de Commissie Late Zwangerschapsafbreking en Levensbeëindiging bij Pasgeborenen over de jaren 2009 en 2010, Ministerie van Volksgezondheid, Welzijn en Sport, p. 18 [Combined annual report of Central committee of experts on late-term abortion and termination of infants over the years 2009 and 2010]

The Dutch government announced that it would review this rule, since certain physicians argued that prevention of future suffering was part of their job.[29] To date, the most recent attempt to liberalize the Dutch rules for termination of life in infants has not been achieved.

How Many Infants Are Involved?

How often does active euthanasia of infants occur in the Netherlands? The most reliable answer is provided by the regular surveys of end-of-life decisions made by physicians. In 2005 the decision to forego pointless medical treatment was made for an estimated seventy infants under the age of one, after which their unavoidable death was accelerated by administering medication for the express purpose of hastening the end of life.[30] Since the discussions of the 1990s many physicians see this as 'assisted dying' rather than 'termination of life'. However, from a legal perspective there is no such thing as 'assisted dying' and it falls under termination of life.[31]

Moreover, in 2005 the lives of approximately ten infants, children who could have survived without medical treatment, were intentionally ended. These children had not been given up by foregoing necessary treatment; their lives were ended on the assumption that they would otherwise suffer severely.[32] This is the group that the Groningen Protocol targets.

Of all the cases of child euthanasia in any year, on average only three are reported to the authorities.[33] Since the *Central Committee of Experts* on late-term abortion and termination of infants was set up in

---

29   Standpunt evaluatie Regeling late zwangerschapsafbreking en levensbeëindiging bij pasgeborenen, 10 juli 2014 [Position Evaluation of Regulation on late-term abortion and termination of infants, July 10 2014]

30   Onwuteaka-Philipsen et al., op.cit.

31   Alex Bood, op.cit.

32   Onwuteaka-Philipsen et al., op. cit., p. 122

33   A.A.E. Verhagen, J.J. Sol, O.F. Brouwer, P.J. Sauer, Actieve levensbeëindiging bij pasgeborenen in Nederland; analyse van alle 22 meldingen uit 1997/'04, *Nederlands Tijdschrift voor Geneeskunde* 2005; 149, p. 186 [Active termination of life in newborns in the Netherlands; an analysis of all 22 reported cases 1997-2004]

2006 to review life termination in newborns, only one case has been reported.[34] It is suspected that the lives of newborns are terminated more often, but these are neither reported nor reviewed.[35]

Pediatricians have indicated to the review committee that they suspect euthanasia occurs less frequently than before. Because of the increased use of ultrasound imaging for women who are twenty weeks pregnant, late-term abortion is chosen more often, which means termination of life after the child is born is less frequent. Children with spina bifida in particular seem to be born only if the parents are determined to let them live.

The one reported case of life termination in a newborn met the requirements of the Groningen Protocol. It concerned a newborn with *epidermolysis bullosa*, a very serious skin disorder. The review committee described that the child suffered from increasing blistering of the skin and skin lesions. Care, even changing diapers, was painful. The child drank less and less and deteriorated. "Initially the child was kept comfortable with the pain relief medication and sedation, except for some personal care moments. He also showed development. He responded well to his parents, followed movement with his eyes and he smiled. However, the child continued to lose weight and it became increasingly difficult to keep him comfortable. He broke through the medication more and more often. In addition his condition weakened to such an extent that he barely opened his eyes and the intake of medication became more and more problematic."

"The father started expressing his wish for active euthanasia three weeks and one day after the birth of his child, during the first conversation

---

34 Gecombineerd Jaarverslag van de Commissie Late Zwangerschapsafbreking en Levens-beëindiging bij Pasgeborenen over de jaren 2009 en 2010, Ministerie van Volksgezond-heid, Welzijn en Sport [Combined 2009-2010 annual report of the Commission for the Acceptability of Life Terminating Action]

35 For more information on lack of notifications of termination of life in newborns and the probability that it is still happening: L.M.H. Bongers, Een beschermwaardig leven. De meerwaarde van de centrale deskundigencommissie rond het levensbeëindigend handelen bij ernstig gehandicapte pasgeborenen, Tilburg, Celsus, 2008, p. 106-107 [A life worth protecting. The added value of the central expert committee for life-terminating action in severely disabled newborns]

with the physician after the baby was readmitted to hospital X. He felt his child was suffering unbearably. At that moment the mother indicated she would prefer to have her child slip away by administering pain medication. She did not support active termination of life."[36] "Eight weeks and six days after the birth of the child she indicated that she now also leaned towards active euthanasia, but that she was in a dilemma. Ten weeks and one day after the birth of their child both parents (finally) expressed consistently and with conviction the wish for active termination of life. It had not been possible to make the child comfortable for about ten days, even with increasingly higher doses of pain medication and sedation."

They then requested active euthanasia for their child, the Expert Committee stated in its annual report. "This was a consistent and well-considered request. Given the hopeless nature of the situation in combination with the unbearable suffering of the child, the physician complied with the request."

The committee concluded that the requirements of due care were met in the only case reported to them. The PPS decided not to prosecute.

Little real debate exists in the Netherlands on active euthanasia in newborns and infants. Most people do not know any details, but simply assume that it is safely regulated. The media, if they take notice of the subject at all, often bring distinctly positive news.

MOVIE: *If We Knew* – The Documentary We Get to See

In 2008 the Dutch public broadcasting service aired the documentary *If We Knew* [*Als we het zouden weten*], which was filmed in the NICU of the University Medical Center Groningen, where the Groningen Protocol was developed. The head of this department is the well-known pediatrician Eduard Verhagen.

The film, by Peter Lataster and Petra Lataster Czisch, shows the distress of parents who gradually realize that their baby will not survive, and the happiness of parents who can leave

---

36   See advice 2009LP01, www.lzalp.nl/adviezen

the ward with their child in an incubator on wheels.

The discussions among physicians and between physicians and parents about the question whether a child can or should be treated are shown extensively. It is remarkable that two physicians from the Groningen team state they are against active termination of life.

The documentary covers the case of an extremely premature child. The Groningen physicians have started treatment. Complications develop, so the prognosis for the child becomes bleaker. In the documentary, Verhagen says to his colleagues: "Had we known about these complications in advance, we would not have started treatment." He concludes: "Now the chance of survival is extremely small and if the child does survive, the way it will survive will probably be exceptionally difficult." Eventually this baby dies.

Two doctors say the concepts of 'livable life' and 'dignified life' help them through the difficult decision whether a baby should be saved. The film-makers do not ask what these concepts entail. Apparently they believe in a criterion that determines whether life is meaningful: it must be 'livable' or 'dignified'. But how is this defined? And who gets to determine that? Can healthy people decide which people with a disability would be better off dead? The film-makers do not ask.

The film-makers do not show whether the physician is allowed to expedite the death of the child by terminating its life once further treatment is considered futile. Verhagen explains that a child whose treatment is discontinued dies a natural death. He does not address the question whether the physician can hasten the imminent death. He does not say whether it is acceptable in that case to actually call it a 'natural death'. The documentary makers did not probe further.

In such cases many physicians like Verhagen, speak of 'accepted medical practice'. Lawyers, however, say that whenever a physician causes a person's death, even when that death was imminent, it is active termination of life.[37] Jurists and

---

37   See, among others, Alex Bood, op. cit.

physicians are talking at cross-purposes here. This is a controversy the documentary did not address.

There is an even larger question that would have been very appropriate to ask here in the very hospital where the Groningen Protocol was established. "Is it acceptable to end the life of a newborn who can survive without intensive medical treatment because the child suffers severely?" This question is virtually ignored in the documentary.

In the documentary, pediatrician Verhagen states that these cases are "very rare and have not occurred in the UMCG since 2007." However, publicity for the documentary *If We Knew* did create the impression that it would address the controversy surrounding the Groningen Protocol. The cover of the DVD, which is also intended for the international market, states: "In 2005 religious groups in Italy and the US accused Dutch pediatricians of using Nazi methods and killing prematurely born babies because of their disabilities." On Holland Doc, a website of the Dutch public broadcasting service, we read this about this film: "Dutch pediatricians are the only ones in the world who have the courage to speak out publicly about this sensitive issue. And not everyone thanks them for it. The so-called "Groningen Protocol" in which pediatrician Eduard Verhagen has established guidelines that can be applied in cases of active euthanasia, caused serious commotion. A group of pediatricians of the UMC Groningen was denounced in the American and Italian media. They were reproached for ending the treatment of premature but viable infants for no reason. One American columnist wrote: "Dr. Mengele is alive and he lives in Holland."

This criticism concerns the Groningen Protocol, that is, the active termination of life of severely ill or disabled newborns who could have survived without intensive care. This theme was not addressed in the film. So the criticism from abroad is used to arouse the public's interest for the film, without showing the controversy that the critics were responding to. Termination of life in ill or disabled newborns was not discussed in the documentary. Viewers would probably wonder what these foreign critics were so worked up about: the documentary makers sidestepped the entire issue that generated the criticism.

This is not unusual in the Netherlands. Foreign criticism is not taken seriously and is defused by reporting it in a greatly exaggerated way.

"As a piece of propaganda the film *If We Knew* is a great success," said Jan Franssen of BOSK, the Dutch patient organization for people with physical disabilities and their parents. "Everything is portrayed with integrity, but we never see the real obstacle, the sting in the discussion."

In 2008 this film won the Dutch *Beeld en Geluid* Award, an important television award for the most appreciated television production. The judges wrote: "It is a documentary filmed up close and personal, in which the makers have not taken a position with regard to their subject."

Difference Of Opinion Between Hospitals

In the Netherlands, the discussion was not completely without conflict. While courts, prosecutors and government continued on the road of termination of life for ever-expanding groups, physicians appeared to be moving towards more restraint.

Dutch pediatricians in the early 2000's seemed less inclined towards euthanasia than in the 1990s. In the mid-1990's, a majority of surveyed pediatricians reported either having ended the life of an infant, or being able to imagine doing so. Ten years later, sixty percent of the pediatricians indicated that active termination of life in newborns was out of the question.[38] The pediatricians remain divided, but the number of those who have convinced the court, PPS and ultimately also the government, that euthanasia can be acceptable in certain situations, is getting smaller and may now be a shrinking minority.

---

38   These data are taken from the repeated surveys of end-of-life decisions of physicians. See G. van der Wal and P.J. van der Maas, *Euthanasie en andere medische beslissingen rond het levenseinde* [Euthanasia and other medical end-of-life decisions], Den Haag, SDU uitgevers, 1996, p. 187; and B.D. Onwuteaka-Philipsen, J.K.M. Gevers and A. van der Heide et al., *Evaluatie wet toetsing levensbeëindiging op verzoek en hulp bij zelfdoding* [Evaluation of the Dutch Euthanasia Act of 2002], Den Haag, ZonMW, 2007, p. 112

Furthermore, some pediatricians question the term 'hopeless and unbearable suffering'. It is a vague term, they argue, which brings a random quality to decisions on euthanasia in newborns. Their concerns were raised by a study of 22 cases of infant euthanasia (Verhagen et.al. 2005). All 22 babies, reported to have been euthanized between 1997 and 2004, had serious forms of spina bifida.[39] According to the physicians who terminated these lives, all 22 babies suffered 'hopelessly and unbearably'.

This satisfied the main legal criterion, but left more experienced observers unconvinced. What roused their curiosity, wrote Rotterdam pediatric surgeon de Jong, clinical ethicist Kompanje and neurologists Arts and Rotteveel,[40] was that babies with spina bifida are not in pain at all. Besides, any pain is easily treated with medication. Apparently, these critics concluded, something else was going on. These twenty-two babies' lives were terminated, not because of any pain, but because they faced a life of serious disability.

The treating physicians who ended the lives of these twenty-two infants applied a wide definition of 'hopeless and unbearable suffering', not limited to pain alone. Also mentioned were a limited ability to live independently and a heavy dependency on medical services in the future. Moreover, in thirteen of the twenty-two cases the prognosis of a long life was an argument to opt for euthanasia: the physicians reasoned that a long life of disability would increase suffering. The prognosis of a life with disabilities was actually used to defend the euthanizing of these thirteen infants.

That is wrong, argued Kompanje, de Jong et.al. (2005) who spoke out against it. The question whether a severe disability is identical with

---

39   A.A.E. Verhagen, J.J. Sol, O.F. Brouwer and P.J. Sauer, Actieve levensbeëindiging bij pasgeborenen in Nederland; analyse van alle 22 meldingen uit 1997/2004, *Nederlands Tijdschrift voor Geneeskunde* 2005; 149: p. 183-188 [Active termination of life in newborns in the Netherlands]

40   E.J.O. Kompanje, T.H.R. de Jong, W.F.M. Arts, J.J. Rotteveel, Problematische basis voor 'uitzichtloos en ondraaglijk lijden' als criterium voor actieve levensbeëindiging bij pasgeborenen met spina bifida, *Nederlands Tijdschrift voor Geneeskunde* 2005; 149: p. 2067-2069 [Problematical basis for 'hopeless and unbearable suffering' as a criterion for active euthanasia in newborns with spina bifida]

'hopeless and unbearable suffering' is better answered by the patients in question when they are a little older. "Then we see that many feel they live meaningful lives, despite their sometimes very serious disabilities" (Kompanje, deJong et al. 2005). "Moreover, the quality of life of children, even with serious forms of spina bifida, is not solely determined by the severity of their disability, but also to a significant degree (...) by the hope parents instill in their children." Erwin Kompanje, ethicist at the Erasmus University Medical Center in Rotterdam, stated that the happiness of a disabled infant depends on its family: "You need someone who believes in you."

After their critical article was published, the father of one of the twenty-two euthanized infants sent an email to the authors telling them they "over-simplified" the issue. This father had wanted to spare his son suffering. In the ensuing contact, the father emailed a picture of his son, taken one hour before his life was to be ended. "He is drinking a bottle in the picture!" said Kompanje. "A child in distress will not drink a bottle quietly. But the parents depend on what the doctor tells them."[41]

The information given to parents of babies with spina bifida in Rotterdam is very different from the information given at Groningen. Said Kompanje: "Here at the Erasmus Medical center we have never performed euthanasia on a baby with spina bifida. We do not see it as a situation of necessity, because we can easily relieve any pain. I am all for active termination of life in the case of acute, actual and untreatable suffering. But two paralyzed legs? No, that is no reason to end a life."

'Hopeless and unbearable suffering' has proven to be a vague term that can be interpreted differently in different hospitals. Without their knowing it, the parents' decision to go to a specific hospital may have deadly consequences for their child.

The critics from the Rotterdam Erasmus Medical Center are emphatic that the vague term has far-reaching consequences from a legal perspective. The Public Prosecution Service will take the physician at his word

---

41 See *The Short Life Of Cas* p. 47

when he claims a 'situation of hopeless and unbearable suffering'. In all twenty-two cases of active euthanasia of a newborn that were reported to the Dutch authorities between 1997 and 2004, the PPS decided not to prosecute because the criteria for 'termination of life' in newborns were supposedly met. The most important of these criteria is that there must have been 'hopeless and unbearable suffering'. Yet the PPS does not check whether there actually was such suffering; it only checks whether the physician refers to it. If he does, the PPS believes him, and there is no further examination of the vague concept. "In this kind of dialogue the physician's assessment proves to be the deciding factor and there is no further review as such," according to clinical ethicist Kompanje, neurosurgeon de Jong and pediatric neurologists Arts and Rotteveel (2005).

Because physicians have a certain degree of freedom to determine whether there exists a situation of "hopeless and unbearable suffering" and to initiate euthanasia, there are differences between hospitals. The Rotterdam Erasmus Medical Center does not apply euthanasia for babies with spina bifida. The University Medical Center Utrecht confirms that there were ten instances of active euthanasia of infants with spina bifida between 1997 and 2004, or almost half of the cases in the Netherlands.

In the opinion of the committee that reviewed termination of life in newborns, this could not be allowed to continue. The hospitals would be required to strive for more consensus. The committee consulted with physicians in 2008 – 2010. They managed to reach agreement on the question as to when a child with spina bifida should be treated and when foregoing treatment is the preferable option. They could not, however, agree on what to do once the decision is made not to treat a child with spina bifida. Is it better to wait until death occurs naturally, or is active euthanasia an acceptable option? "The discussion focuses on the question whether you only look at pain, or do you also take into consideration the futility of the life," the committee reported.[42]

---

42   Gecombineerd Jaarverslag van de Commissie Late Zwangerschapsafbreking en Levensbeëindiging bij Pasgeborenen over de jaren 2009 en 2010, Ministerie van Volksgezondheid, Welzijn en Sport, p.7 [Combined 2009-2010 annual report of the Commission for the Acceptability of Life Terminating Action]

Incidentally, the entire above discussion about life and death of babies with spina bifida is exceptional. Most cases of termination of life in newborns are never discussed by the PPS or the review committee – because they are not reported. The twenty-two cases examined by Verhagen et al. (2005) were all reported in the seven and a half years between January 1997 and June 2004. Based on surveys among physicians it is actually assumed that during a four-month period in 2001 alone, the lives of thirty-two infants under the age of one were ended by administering a drug for this explicit purpose.[43]

The public plan for the future is to convince physicians to report any instance of euthanasia of an infant to the Special Expert Committee. However, this does not totally convince the critics in Rotterdam. If such a committee is to have any significance, then at least let it render its judgment before the life of the infant is ended rather than afterwards.[44]

Lawyers Also Have Critical Comments

A few Dutch jurists also asked critical questions about 'termination of life' in newborns. Jo Dorscheidt, assistant professor of Health Law, has investigated whether the deliberate ending of life in newborns is in violation of the ban on discrimination of the disabled.[45] He pointed out that as soon as a doctor says a baby suffers hopelessly and unbearably, the PPS believes the doctor and does not pursue the matter. Nobody examines whether the baby that was killed actually did suffer hopelessly and unbearably. This jurist's concerned is that life is terminated, not because the child suffers severely, but because it is has a disability.

---

43 Het levenseinde in de medische praktijk. Resultaten sterfgevallenonderzoek 2001, Voorburg/Heerlen, Centraal Bureau voor de Statistiek, 2003, p. 32 [The end of life in medical practice]

44 T.H.R. de Jong, E. van Lindert, E.J.O. Kompanje, J.J. Rotteveel, Laten sterven of doen sterven? Palliatieve zorg voldoet bij pasgeborenen met onbehandelbare spina bifida, *Medisch Contact* 61, 2006, p. 669-671 [Let die or cause to die? Palliative care suffices in newborns with untreatable spina bifida]

45 J.H.H.M. Dorscheidt, Levensbeëindiging bij gehandicapte pasgeborenen. Strijdig met het anti-discriminatiebeginsel? Dissertatie RU Groningen, Sdu, Den Haag, 2006, p. 109-110 [Termination of life in disabled newborns. Compatible with the Principle of Non-Discrimination?].

According to international agreements, this kind of discrimination would be wrong. The first UN human rights instrument that ruled out discrimination on the basis of disability, the *International Convention on the Rights of the Child* (ICRC), expressly forbade such discrimination. It has been in force in the Netherlands since March 1995. "It is remarkable that the prevalent analyses of the legal aspects of ending the life of disabled infants barely mention the human rights perspective." The main issue of the Groningen protocol seems to be the seriousness of the newborn's disabilities, while forgetting that a disabled newborn has basic rights, such as the right to life and the right to healthcare.

Dorscheidt (2006) also called attention to the less than orderly way of thinking about euthanasia. Many words have been used, but no real weighing of pros and cons has taken place. Therefore, no logical conclusion can be reached. "It is striking that the opinions that consider ending damaged newborn life acceptable only pay lip service to the fundamental rights of the young disabled child. Arguments to defend such positions generally do no more than mention the rights of the child, in particular the right to life." Dorscheidt further argued that presumptions of the wishes of the child and presumptions of the best interest of the child "are generally considered sufficient justification for the limitation of the child's right to life."[46]

The physicians' thinking is often at odds with the law, Dorscheidt stated. In their report *To Act or Not?*, the pediatricians argued that "even in situations in which in all fairness it is still possible to speak of human life," life-terminating action is not automatically contrary to the right to life guaranteed in the *European Convention on Human Rights*.

Dorscheidt objected in the strongest possible terms. "The first problem is the formulated principle 'even in situations in which in all fairness it is still possible to speak of human life'. From a legal perspective every human individual born alive is considered 'human life'. This life is part of the community of legal persons, and as a legal subject it is due all legal protection, regardless of his level of existence." It is definitely

---

[46]   Ibid., p.65

conceivable that people, because of their suffering, voluntarily give up the right to life and prefer to die. Yet they can only do this voluntarily; only voluntary euthanasia is possible. For human rights are inalienable, Dorscheidt argued. No physician can judge on behalf of a newborn that he is better off dead.[47]

Dorscheidt did not completely exclude termination of life without request. He wanted it justified. Furthermore, this justification must never discriminate against people with a disability. Making, or letting, a child die just because of the simple fact that it had a condition would clearly be discrimination. A child with Down syndrome also has rights; it would be discrimination to let this child die merely because of its condition, according to Dorscheidt. An objective justification to make termination of life acceptable should (1) always be concrete, and (2) always relate to the particular child. He calls for jurists and physicians, together, to ask more questions and think the matter through more profoundly

Dorscheidt insists that the standards of legal clarity must apply. If a physician refused treatment because in his opinion it is 'medically futile', we should be told exactly *why* the treatment is medically point-less. If the physician refers to 'poor quality of life', this is too vague for legal standards. If the physician refers to 'limited communication possibilities of the child', Dorscheidt responds that, in court, poor communicative possibilities are no reason to end a life.

Health lawyer and Philosophy of Law professor Martin Buijsen has expressed surprise that State Secretary Ross-van Dorp and Minister Donner listed 'independence' as a criterion for life termination in infants in the Dutch Second Chamber: "The health situation of the child in those cases offers absolutely no prospect of any kind of independent life," according to Ross-van Dorp and Donner.[48] However, the law does not

---

47   Ibid., p. 142-143

48   Kamerstukken II 2005/06, 30300, XVI, nr. 90, p.3-4, geciteerd in M.A.J.M. Buijsen, Impliciete keuzes en verhulde waardeoordelen: het kabinetsvoorstel Actieve levensbeëindiging bij ernstig lijdende pasgeborenen, Nederlands Juristenblad (2006) 15: 832-839 [Implicit decisions and veiled value judgments: the parliamentary proposal Active termination of life in severely suffering newborns]

specify that only self-reliant persons are allowed to live, says Buijsen. Human rights apply to all who are born from people, including those who will never be able to live independently. By saying that inadequate self-reliance is a criterion for termination of life, the government, in very veiled terms, has executed a value judgment. "This value judgment is not expressed, or defended, but it appears that medical professionals (and parents) are permitted to apply it in practice."[49]

Buijsen, while working at the Rotterdam Erasmus Medical Center, wrote this critical article at the request of BOSK, the Dutch patient organization for people with physical disabilities and their parents. BOSK protects the interests of, among others, people with spina bifida. BOSK has been one of the few organizations in the Netherlands to ask critical questions about the issue whether the ending of life in disabled newborns is allowed. It is, perhaps, no coincidence that in the Hague, the political center of the Netherlands, there was almost no discussion.

Buijsen (2005) stated that the Dutch government has tried to depoliticize the discussion on termination of the lives of newborns with disabilities. It acted as if, from a political point of view, there was nothing to discuss and it was fine to leave everything to the experts. The second cabinet under Prime Minister Balkenende, supported in parliament by a coalition of the Christian Democrats (CDA), right-wing liberals (VVD) and left-wing liberals (D66), therefore only talked about 'procedures' during the years that the Groningen Protocol was being formulated. The fundamental decisions that led the government to consider deliberate termination of life infants with disabilities "are barely if at all justified," according to Buijsen.

There is a possibility that this will cause a problem for the Netherlands in the international arena. The Netherlands has signed the *International Covenant on Civil and Political Rights* (ICCPR), among other things. In August 2001 the *UN Human Rights Committee* that investigates compliance with this Covenant lashed out at the Netherlands: "The Committee is gravely concerned at reports that new-born

---

49   Buijsen, op. cit., p. 839

handicapped infants have had their lives ended by medical personnel."
The Committee called this a violation of the right to life, as defined in
the covenant, and requested the Dutch government to inform the UN
Committee on the number of such cases and on the results of court proceedings following from these cases.[50]

There appears to be little chance of that happening. Since that time, no
physician who has ended the life of a newborn has ever appeared before a
Dutch court, although studies of medical end-of-life decisions show that
termination of life in newborn infants does in fact still take place.

CONTEXT: *Eduard Verhagen* and the Groningen Protocol

"Openness and transparency," says the pediatrician of
the University Medical Center Groningen Eduard Verhagen,
"those are the key words." Verhagen, who spoke clearly, deliberately and confidently, had a leading role in formulating
the Groningen Protocol.

"The protocol was formulated because of a little girl with
blister disease," a serious condition in which the skin of the
child does not function properly. "The parents actually beat us
to it; they had already searched the internet when we wanted
to tell them the poor prognosis, and they had come to the
conclusion on their own that euthanasia would be in the best
interest of their child." But because the law prohibited termination of life without request, Verhagen and his colleagues
refused. "The child died several months later, of pneumonia.
In retrospect we wondered whether it would have been better to have shortened her suffering." Things would have to be
different from then on.

Because Verhagen wanted to be upfront and not act in se-
crecy, he needed to reach public agreements. That is how the
Groningen Protocol came into being.

According to Verhagen, the Groningen Protocol only applies to that group of newborns who could survive outside

---

50 Concluding observations of the Human Rights Committee: Netherlands. 27/08/2001.
CCPR/CO/72/NET

the NICU, but are suffering severely. There are very few such cases each year. Generally, these children do not need mechanical ventilation. In these cases, discontinuing treatment to cause the desired death is not possible. Verhagen: "There is nothing to discontinue there."

The second group of children is much more common – those newborns who do depend on mechanical ventilation and other types of intensive care. If the decision is made that it is better for them to die, because they would have very poor quality of life, their treatment can be discontinued. "Further treatment is possible, but sometimes the decision is made not to continue." Often a child dies quickly after the treatment is stopped or the ventilator is disconnected. If dying takes too long, some pediatricians will hasten the child's passing. "The latter is part of accepted medical practice," according to Verhagen. It therefore does not fall under the Groningen Protocol.

Finally, there is the third and largest group of children who die in the NICU. These are children for whom treatment is futile and who will inevitably die. No controversy there.

The first two groups of infants could possibly survive, but the decision is made for them that it is better to die. The physicians base this decision on the anticipated quality of life of the child.

Is the term "quality of life" not too vague? Verhagen: "What I say is: come and see, then you'll know." In the NICU he presents an extremely premature baby girl. "She has already been on a ventilator for three months." Since artificial respiration damages the lungs, the situation becomes bleaker as the respiration continues. What is making the girl so sick that she needs artificial respiration is not clear. "The question now is: can she still make it, and if she does, is there a chance of a meaningful life, or will she be a vegetable?"

Should the decision be made to let this girl die, no active termination of life will be required. Due to her bad lungs Verhagen expects her to die within ten minutes after the ventilator is shut down. Medication can prevent suffering in those last minutes of her life.

Termination of life can be the best option not only for newborn infants who are suffering now. In 2007 Verhagen suggested considering termination of life in the case of anticipated future suffering. This proposal was made by the Pediatrician, Ethics and Law Commission of the Dutch Pediatric Association, of which Verhagen is a member.

These physicians named two remarkable criteria to judge that the infant's future life will be too hard. First, they mention an anticipated long life expectancy as a criterion for termination of life: in this case the suffering as a result of the illness lasts too long. Second, two paragraphs later they write that an anticipated short life expectancy can be a criterion to end the life of a newborn infant.[51]

Is there no contradiction in putting forward both a long and short life expectancy as reasons for termination of life? "No, the arguments do not contradict each other. They complement each other," says Verhagen. "The point is that the situation of the child is the deciding factor.

CONTEXT: *BOSK – "Right To Life Is The Starting Point"*

"A prognosis is only a prognosis, it does not say anything about a child's will to live," says Johannes Verheijden of BOSK, the Dutch patient organization for people with physical disabilities and their parents. Physicians who present a poor prognosis are not always right. Physicians, say Verheijden, have limited predictive powers regarding how a child born with spina bifida will fare.

And yet the influence of the physician's prognosis is considerable: it is the deciding factor in whether a child will be treated or not. The result is life, or death. This influence increases when the physician's prognosis is formulated to push the parents in a particular direction. Jan Franssen, also of

---

51 A.A.E. Verhagen, M.A.H.B.M. van der Hoeven, J.B. van Goudoever, M.C. de Vries, A.Y.N. Schouten-van Meeteren, M.J.I.J. Alberts, Uitzichtloos en ondraaglijk lijden en actieve levensbeëindiging bij pasgeborenen, *Nederlands Tijdschrift voor Geneeskunde* 2007; 151: p. 1474-1477, zie p. 1476 [Hopeless and unbearable suffering and active termination of life in newborns]

BOSK: "It makes a difference whether the doctor says: "Your child will be confined to a wheelchair" or "Your child will have mobility with a wheelchair.""

Sometimes it is better not to decide immediately for or against treatment on the basis of a prognosis. Wait to see if the child shows a desire to live, says Franssen. "The child will show you whether it is a fighter and wants to live or not." By looking at what the child shows before deciding to start treatment or not, the decision is based not only on what the medical manual prescribes, but also on the impression that parents get from their child.

When it is decided to forego treatment, the question is sometimes asked whether active termination of life should be applied. For BOSK the right to life is the starting point. At present physicians have too much power to decide on termination of life, according to BOSK. That is why the organization wants a compulsory review by an independent organization of a decision to actively terminate a life before it is carried out.

To prove that it is possible to grow up with spina bifida, BOSK made a poster portraying 150 adults who were born with this condition. "That made an impression," Verheijden recounts. "At the time the decision was made for all these people to start treatment. Now they are adults, they work, they participate in society."

CONTEXT: *The Short Life Of Cas, Born With Spina Bifida*

"My wife at the time was pregnant and she noticed it first. "I'm not happy," she said, "he doesn't kick me as much as the first one did." Three weeks before the baby was due, an ultrasound revealed spina bifida." Dirk Paardekoper is talking about his second son, Cas. "The doctors said there might be a problem with his legs or his mind, and that he could be incontinent." The parents started thinking it would be a good idea to have the nursery on the ground floor. "We were thinking in terms of solutions, to keep us from going crazy."

On Thursday February 7 2003 Cas was born at the Groningen University Hospital (UMCG). Dirk Paardekooper: "I was a bit apprehensive beforehand, but when I saw him I immediately fell in love." He had contractures in his legs and there was a large cyst at the base of his spine, where it hadn't closed properly.

"Our perspective at the time was: a couple of months of treatment in the hospital and then we'll take it from there. But on the first day the doctors told us if his heart stops they would rather not resuscitate, because then he will have even more problems." This sounded like a reasonable argument. On the second day the doctors said the same about his lungs. So we made the same decision about his lungs, Cas would not be put on a ventilator. The doctor looked more worried every day. And we became more stressed every day. But of course we continued to sing songs, tell stories and hug him."

"On Sunday we let his big brother come over for the first time, he was six years old then. After that he visited almost every day."

"On Tuesday the doctor came and said: "We recommend not to treat and to let him die. The opening is located very low on his back, which means it is not likely he will ever be able to sit upright and he would probably have to live in an institution his entire life," Dirk Paardekooper recounts. It was too early for the doctors to tell whether Cas was also affected mentally. But if he survived the parents should hope that he was, the doctor said, because then he would not be aware of his limited abilities compared to the people around him. "It was very harsh but also very honest of them to say that."

"What was very important to us was that he would be in a lot of pain. His spine was going to grow crooked and because his torso would collapse he would also have trouble breathing."

Now the parents had to decide whether they agreed with the doctors. The prognosis was that Cas could survive, he could live to be sixty. His father remembers trying to arrive at a decision: "Sixty years, in so much pain, confined to a bed, with all those disabilities. He wouldn't be able to stay at home, he would have to live in an institution and we would visit once or a few times a week."

The parents questioned whether they could cope with this and realized they could not. "No, we can't bear it, so it is unfair to ask our child to bear it," Dirk Paardekooper and his wife concluded. "But emotionally it is a different story: your instinct as a parent is to hold him and take him home." As his father is still convinced today, this was not in the best interest of Cas. "It was an impossible choice and we made the least bad decision."

"I was in the shower and I prayed: God, if this is the wrong decision please make the water turn red. Because this was the hardest decision of my life."

The doctors told us about parents who had made the opposite decision, and who now dared to admit only in the doctor's office that it had been the wrong decision.

On Wednesday afternoon Cas was given pain medication that immediately put him into a coma. The doctor told us that at some point his heart would be unable to keep beating; this could take anywhere from a few hours up to months. "Then we said: A few months – we can't handle that."

Dirk Paardekooper recounts how his then wife and he saw their son struggle to breathe. "Every now and then his lips would turn blue and his breathing would slow down. So we told him: "It's okay to go, Cas, go back to the source." But then he would suddenly take a deep breath."

"They had told us: "If you can't cope with it, then termination of life is an option." That night we said: "No we can't take any more. Four weeks of incredible stress from the moment of the ultrasound, we are exhausted." On Wednesday February 12 at 9:45 PM the doctor gave Cas an injection, fifteen minutes later he passed away. For privacy reasons, the hospital (UMCG) has declined to comment on this case.

"Before he went into a coma, he was a happy, big, ten-pound baby. I have a picture of him leaning on his little arms. He had great upper body strength."

The morning after Cas died the doctor talked to the parents

again. "You have made the right decision," she said. But it didn't feel like it," Dirk Paardekooper explains. "Then we sent for his big brother, and his grandmother, and we explained to him that Cas was very ill and that the doctors couldn't make him better. You can't explain to a six-year-old that it involved an ethical dilemma and that you let them cause the death of his baby brother."

"Does this mean that we made the wrong decision?" Dirk Paardekooper wondered when doctors from the Rotterdam Erasmus University Medical Centre voiced their criticism. In their view termination of life was unnecessary in this and similar cases of babies born with spina bifida, because they were not in pain. "Groningen could set our minds at ease on this point. They said that Cas had been in pain. And they also felt that the prognosis for his quality of life was important. Rotterdam takes an extremely formal position here: when there is no or very little pain you are not allowed to do anything."

He thinks the public debate between pediatricians is a good thing. However, he has a big problem with the differences between hospitals regarding babies like Cas. "In one hospital treatment is started automatically based on its religious affiliation, the next hospital leaves it up to the parents to decide. A decision of this magnitude should be made by the parents."

Chapter 4

New Bones Of Contention

After the Euthanasia Act

Those who think that the 2002 euthanasia law put an end to the discussion on termination of life are mistaken. On the contrary, the advent of the law that allowed the killing of people in specific situations has launched numerous controversial issues.

The Dutch right-to-die association NVVE set itself some new goals. First, it changed its name from *Dutch Association for Voluntary Euthanasia* to *Dutch Association for a Voluntary End to Life*, a more comprehensive concept. Since February 2008 the goal of the NVVE is to make "a chosen end of life" possible for people with dementia, mentally ill people, and people who are old and tired of life. Because their competence is in question, the Euthanasia Act often does not cover people in the first two categories. NVVE's most striking proposal is to help a third group of people to commit suicide: those who are over the age of seventy and tired of life, but not ill.[52] The Euthanasia Act does not yet cover this group, because there is no 'hopeless and unbearable suffering'. To

---

[52] NVVE, *Perspectieven op waardig sterven*, Amsterdam, 2008, p. 24 [Perspectives on dying with dignity]

change this, the NVVE, together with the Dutch citizens' action group Of One's Own Free Will [Uit Vrije Wil] is fighting to amend the law.

In addition, some physicians argue that the Dutch euthanasia law is too strict to offer a solution for severely suffering children. They argue that it should also be possible to end the life of children under the age of twelve. Today these children are still outside the scope of the euthanasia act because they are not legally competent to consent. Each of these three controversial proposals will be explored below.

Mobile Euthanasia Teams

Every year hundreds of patients, believing that the Euthanasia Act had created new rights, are disappointed as doctors reject or postpone their plans. The *Dutch Association for a Voluntary End to Life*, NVVE opened an end-of-life-clinic in The Hague in 2012; patients can go there for euthanasia or physician-assisted suicide. The clinic also has mobile teams that drive around the country to help people die at home. This end-of-life clinic and its mobile teams bridge the gap between the patients' expectations and the legal reality. Most people in The Netherlands believe that they are entitled to euthanasia or physician assisted suicide, but the Euthanasia Act gives the right to comply or reject such a request to the physicians alone. Many physicians will only help euthanize patients they know personally. NVVE contends that patients whose doctors refuse to assist them have a problem. Since 2012, they can turn to the end-of-life-clinic and its mobile teams. However, these are also bound by the law, and consequently cannot comply with every request.

Assisted Suicide For Elderly People Who Are Tired Of Life

"Done with life." Advocates of the latest expansion employ this phrase to refer to elderly people who see no reason to go on living. They long for death, argues NVVE, but if death does not come, the government must assist them.

Citizens' initiative group *Of One's Own Free Will* and the NVVE say they want to give every individual the right to 'decide their own fate'. At the time of writing, 116,871 Dutch citizens have indicated they support changing the law to reach this goal.

Assisted suicide is already permitted under the Dutch Euthanasia Act, but only when carried out by a physician in the case of severe suffering. The step advocated by *Of One's Own Free Will* would drop the requirement for 'hopeless and unbearable suffering' and make assisted suicide an option for people who have reached their seventies and believe they have lived long enough. Authorities should specifically designate certain 'healthcare professionals' to help these people die.

The Dutch parliament expressed little enthusiasm for the bill in early 2011. However, the advocates plan to come back in the future, when the rapidly changing political landscape is more receptive to their cause.

Dutch physicians have not rejected the proposal out of hand, but they did not welcome it either. KNMG, the *Royal Dutch Medical Association*, suggested a compromise. They would regard any minor combination of geriatric afflictions of an elderly person as 'hopeless and unbearable suffering.' Requests for assisted suicide from elderly persons could therefore be met within the boundaries of the Euthanasia Act, without the need for amendments. Some Dutch physicians are already stretching the boundaries of the euthanasia law: when a patient requests to die, the physician can always find a less severe affliction to justify the requested assistance with suicide or euthanasia. Some of these cases have already been approved by the Euthanasia Act review committees.

But Of *One's Own Free Will* demands an amendment to the law: everyone over the age of seventy must be able to obtain euthanasia from specially trained professionals without having to refer to illness as an excuse and without the direct involvement of a physician.

It is questionable whether this plan, if it were to become law, would set clear boundaries for assisted suicide in actual practice. At a meeting of *Of One's Own Free Will* and the Dutch Humanist Association on November 9 2010 in Amsterdam, so many sympathizers attended that a few individuals forgot it was a public gathering. The famous neurobiologist

Dick Swaab, one of the initiators, said: "The age limit is arbitrary. Just between you and me: this age limit was chosen for pragmatic reasons, so we would have a chance to obtain majority support in parliament." It is obvious that it would be difficult to enforce such a limit. Assisted suicide can hardly be punishible in the case of a 68-year-old if it is permissible for a 72-year-old. A likely outcome is that people under the age of seventy who wish to die would also be allowed to ask for help to end their lives.

Another supporter of the amendment who raised questions about whether such assisted suicide can be responsibly regulated is Eugene Sutorius, a well-known Dutch lawyer who has played a major role in the euthanasia movement. At a symposium of the *Dutch Lawyers' Association Pro Vita* (JPV) on January 15 2011 in Rotterdam he explained that it is not easy to find the right name for the group of people that *Of One's Own Free Will* wants to help. 'People who consider their lives complete' is not the right description; 'people who are done with life' is not either; in fact there is no accurate description, Sutorius said. *Of One's Own Free Will* is therefore advocating the possibility to help an indefinable, elusive group of people to commit suicide. However, you cannot determine limits for what you cannot define. The fact that even Sutorius, a lawyer, has trouble coming up with an adequate definition indicates that as soon as it passes into law, the initiative that is now intended only for a small group of elderly people could develop into a vaguely defined right for people to help one another commit suicide.

If this bill were passed into law in the future, the Netherlands would permit non-physicians to assist the suicides of people who are not suffering but still want to die. This could be justified with an appeal to self-determination: who are we to stop another person who wants to die? However, the question not being asked by *Of One's Own Free Will* is whether this will create pressure. Pressure on people to die.

It is no coincidence that *Of One's Own Free Will* consists of cultured, highly educated people who can quietly ponder ending their lives. In the real world, however, there are weak people, bad people, and there are also many good people who occasionally have bad moments. Suppose the law is amended and suicide becomes a respectable option. Suppose you have suffered from mental illness for twenty years. The arguments with your family, the loss of your friends, the looks you get from your neighbors are all daily reminders of the fact that you are unstable, maladjusted at the very least, that you cost society a lot and contribute nothing. What if your children, your neighbors, the last acquaintances who still call you now and then, know "he can die if he wants to." The mere fact that people around you know this will change the relationship you have with them. "You choose to continue living, so you have no right to complain."

Suppose suicide becomes just another option available to free individuals. Imagine you are discharged from the drug rehabilitation clinic for the third time. In less than a week you are using again. Your friends and family have always supported you, but now your problems are driving them to desperation. And you have the option to die: you know it and they know it. In the Netherlands everybody has the right to decide, it's all soundly organized. Perhaps your friends will be open-minded enough to remind you of this option.

There is a real risk that people will no longer be allowed to be troublesome, that pressure will be brought to bear on annoying, ill, maladjusted people to end it all. What starts as self-determination can end as condescension and paternalism.

Even if an individual appears to choose suicide completely voluntarily, even if it does look like the much-romanticized free human being choosing his *freitod* [honorable suicide] there is another consequence that the advocates do not mention. One man's free will affects others. Dutch author and essayist Joost Zwagerman has described what suicide does to those who are left behind. Children whose fathers or mothers die by their own hand frequently also end their own lives, Zwagerman writes.[53] Parental suicide increases the likelihood of their children also committing suicide. So how free is the choice of this child when he chooses to die by his own hand? It happens: families in which not just one, but two members end their own life. Son commits suicide, mother can't cope and follows suit a few days later. Or the reverse: father dies by his own hand, daughter follows him years later.

The advocates of assisted suicide do not take these chains of suicide into consideration. They focus on the individual, who is thought to make decisions totally autonomously, and ignore the people around him. Regardless of whether the environment influences the individual or vice versa, whether the people around him drive the troublesome individual to suicide, or the individual who takes his own life leaves a trail of destruction in his wake and drives others to suicide: the supporters of assisted suicide do not include either type of influencing between people in their considerations. They only see heroic individuals.

Another controversy provoked by the Euthanasia Act is the demand that psychiatric patients should also be able to get help to end their life if they want to.

MOVIE: *Please Let Me Die*

In 2008 Eveline van Dijck, commissioned by the Dutch Humanist Association, made the documentary film *Please Let Me Die* [*Mag ik dood*].

Some years earlier, van Dijck's sister suffered from mental illness and hanged herself. The documentary maker has wondered ever since whether it would have been better had she been able to help her sister end her life, so the suicide did not have to be quite so cruel. On the documentary's website www.magikdood.nl the subject matter of the film is described as follows: *"Please let me die* is about the lack of help for people with a chronic mental illness who wish to die." The word

---

53   Zwagerman, Joost, *Door eigen hand. Zelfmoord en de nabestaanden*, Amsterdam/Antwerpen, de Arbeiderspers, 2005, p. 13 en 36 [By their own hand. Suicide and the people who are left behind.]

'help' in this context means 'help to end their own life'.

There is a gap between the public debate about euthanasia and the legal reality. This film portrays the resulting tension. The general public thinks that the Euthanasia Act established a right to euthanasia or assisted suicide, when it merely protects doctors from investigation. When they demand euthanasia from their physician, they find they cannot force him to comply. Psychiatrists in particular don't like the notion of assisted suicide, because their patient's wish to die may result from his mental illness. The patient is therefore not really capable of making this decision. And without the physician's cooperation there will be no euthanasia – in other words, no self-determination for the mentally ill. Regular citizens are not allowed to assist with suicide in the Netherlands, only physicians are. This makes assisted suicide for people with mental illnesses virtually impossible in practice. The advocates of the possibility of assisted suicide for psychiatric patients are now pressing the Dutch psychiatrists to let go of their reserve.

Back to *Please Let Me Die*. We see the now-deceased sister alive in a shot, her sister Eveline trying to encourage her. "For God's sake, try to hold on." "I don't know how." "Just keep going." Documentary maker Eveline van Dijck: "She has tried her very best to make it work for the past two years. Mainly for us, I think now."

Then the documentary continues with other surviving relatives, who all talk about a husband, wife, son, daughter, brother or sister who took their own life. The documentary maker does not focus on the people who died, who they were or why they wanted to die. She focuses on how they ended their life. Then she says to the relatives: "A modern civilization should not allow that people have to turn to turpentine, or a train." Eveline van Diuck's reasoning appears to be that because of the sometimes gruesome methods of suicide it is better if we help suicidal people kill themselves, so it can be less brutal and lonely.

Marleen van Bijnen, humanistic counselor and staff member at the Dutch Right-to-Die association NVVE agrees: "The

NVVE feels that you should not abandon this very large group... that you should not turn your back on them." In this case "not abandon" or "not turn your back on" means that you help a person with suicidal tendencies to end his life.

This new definition of the word 'help' is used equally euphemistically in the documentary by Eveline van Dijck. "Suppose it was an option... then we can investigate together and at least we would know which medication... I think that would have been a tremendous reassurance for my sister." All the relatives of people who have killed themselves agree. To the people who are interviewed in this documentary 'being able to help' is synonymous with: help with suicide. One person says, for example: "you are better off being an animal. Then you go to the vet ...and then they are put down."

It makes sense that many surviving relatives wonder whether a less brutal form of leaving this life would have been possible. That some also wonder whether the suicide would have been less brutal had they assisted, also makes sense. But it is equally logical to expect that some people wonder the opposite: whether by helping they could have prevented the suicide of their lover, friend or relative. In the documentary we do not hear from this group. Eveline van Dijck lets only those people speak who, like herself and the people who commissioned the film, feel that assisted suicide must be made possible.

Then Els Borst, who helped realize the 2001 Euthanasia Act, appears on the screen. The former Minister of Health (from the left-liberal *Democrat 66* party) explains that her euthanasia act does not exclude the mentally ill. "The psychiatrists must make the subject discussible," says Borst. By 'making discussible' she means that psychiatrists must bring up euthanasia and assisted suicide in their discussions with patients with chronic mental illnesses. In this way the patients understand they are allowed to ask for it. Many physicians erroneously neglect to do this, according to the former Minister of Health.

A debate on this documentary was organized by the Dutch Humanist Association in 2008 in the town of Apeldoorn.

During the debate, NVVE's director Jonquière targeted the psychiatrists who were present, asking why they withhold assisted suicide from their patients, while family doctors do help patients who ask for it: "What is the difference with the family doctor? ... Why can't the treating psychiatrist do it, I don't understand."[54]

The film *Please Let Me Die* does not discuss the possibility that psychiatric patients are influenced in their wish to die – by their illness, their family, or perhaps their doctor. Consider a psychiatrist who, as Els Borst advocates, did bring up euthanasia or assisted suicide to a psychiatric patient. That could be interpreted as a suggestion. A patient might request suicide because the psychiatrist brought it up without being asked. The mere awareness that his family has suffered, perhaps for decades, the consequences of his own mental illness could pressure the patient to choose death. Another possibility is that the mental illness itself can make a person suicidal, which creates doubt whether the choice to kill oneself is really a free choice or a symptom of the disease. The documentary does not ask or answer any question that can raise doubt about whether a psychiatric patient who says he wants to die really makes the decision himself. The film's premise is pure self-determination, a world in which everybody, including a psychiatric patient with suicidal tendencies, is quite capable of making his own decisions with no risk of being influenced by anyone or anything else.

MOVIE: *Before I Forget*

A somewhat similar documentary is *Before I Forget* [*Voor ik het vergeet*], made by Nan Rosens for Dutch public television in 2008. This film is about assisted suicide for people in the early stages of dementia. This documentary was made with the cooperation of, once again, the Dutch Humanist Association, the NVVE, documentary maker Eveline van Dijck and *De Einder*, a foundation that counsels people who want to end their lives.

---

54   Debate June 21 2008; CODA, Apeldoorn

Before I Forget is about Paul van Eerde, a 'veritable bon vivant' who, the moment he is diagnosed with early-stage dementia, starts to think about suicide. His wife quotes her husband: "I will not end up like a zombie with a wet diaper in a wheelchair." As we will see, it is not uncommon to use this 'zombie in a diaper' image to describe people with dementia in the Netherlands. The son articulates his fathers reasons: "He also didn't want to do that to us." The daughter talks about her father's death wish: "That was the father I knew. This immediately turned it into something almost beautiful and tough."

Paul van Eerde discusses his wish to die with his family doctor, who says he is not enthusiastic about assisted suicide. This again demonstrates the limits of the current Dutch euthanasia law: if the physician says no, the patient does not get what he wants. Going to another doctor is not as obvious as one might think – Dutch people generally have a relationship of trust with their family doctors, built up over many years. If the doctor won't help, you really have a problem.

During the spring of 2006 Paul van Eerde mentions his wish to die less frequently. His wife describes the dilemma she feels: she does not want to pressure him to hurry up, but neither should he wait too long. What if he forgets and is no longer able to kill himself? The dementia will continue to get worse. "What really bothers me is that it is hard sometimes to deal with the uncertainty and then I think: just make the decision and do it. But that is caused partly by my fear, my concern, that he will wait so long that he doesn't understand anymore, doesn't want to anymore, can't do it anymore." His daughter also talks about the problem her father is having with deciding the right moment for his intended suicide. She quotes him: "So the moment is going to be a real problem; I can still enjoy life now, but well, I mustn't be too late, because if I am too late, later on, to make the decision, then it won't be possible anymore." In the meantime Van Eerde has turned for help to Ton Vink, a counselor of De Einder, the foundation that helps people who want to end their life. In doing so Vink is operating on the edge of the law.

When Van Eerde experiences another panic attack he decides the moment to end his life is drawing near. His wife quotes him: "We are going on holiday, we are going to have a great holiday and when we get back we will organize everything and set the date." Paul van Eerde has a farewell reception for all his friends. Seeing him say goodbye to his two best friends brings tears to his son's eyes, but Van Eerde doesn't really understand anymore why his son is crying.

The family subsequently retires into the house and then the moment is there. Van Eerde's wife recounts: "When we walked into the bedroom together where everything was prepared, well I had a feeling like, OK we just have to do this now, I had no real sense of what was actually going on, and sometimes I still don't. Then I think: what in heaven's name must he have felt when he dragged himself into that bedroom to take that stuff?' His son says: "My father looked happy and relieved when he had finished eating the mush-like mixture."

However, even though the mush contains a large quantity of drugs Paul van Eerde does not die, he only loses consciousness. In a panic the family approaches the family doctor the next day, but he refuses to come and kill the father. After two days Paul van Eerde dies, the pills did their work after all. The daughter talks about the paradoxical relief she felt then: "It is so totally bizarre that you feel happy instead of sad. He made it. Yes, he did it!"

On the Internet the documentary received many approving reactions. The general tenor of the reactions was that euthanasia is not properly organized in the Netherlands. The documentary was awarded a prize in 2012.

A "debate" about this television documentary was programmed for November 11 2008 in Amsterdam. Not a single opponent of euthanasia for people with dementia was invited. At the request of the moderator, the event started off with a round of applause for the Van Eerde family. "A courageous family," in the words of host Lex Bohlmeijer. Stella Braam, journalist and publicist on Alzheimer's disease, disclosed that her father had suffered from dementia, but his request for euthanasia had come too late. He was already incompetent at the time, so the nursing home physician refused to cooperate. As a daughter she had let the moment pass, perhaps because she loved her father and did not want him to die. So she advised the audience to appoint an 'objective outsider' who will keep an eye on the time so people who become demented don't wait too long to choose death while they are still legally competent.

Lawyer Esther Pans asserted that euthanasia in the case of dementia is allowed in the Netherlands, as long as you are still competent and you can find a physician who is willing to help. To date a significant number of euthanasia cases of people with dementia have been reported to the euthanasia review committees. All have been accepted. Esther Pans: "The possibility exists." Family doctor Sytske van der Meer, who claimed she has twice carried out euthanasia on a person with early-stage dementia confirmed this: "The ball is rolling."

The "debate" about *Before I Forget* notwithstanding, not all physicians cooperate this easily. Euthanasia in early-stage dementia is on the edge of what the law allows. It is also one of the three controversial issues that the NVVE and the Humanist Association have resolutely been campaigning for since 2008. Physician Petra de Jong, director of NVVE, insists that physicians should be subject to disciplinary action if they refuse to provide euthanasia themselves or to refer the patient to a physician who would. This would compel the physicians to be more cooperative.

Already, some physicians are finding room within the Euthanasia Act to provide euthanasia and assisted suicide for people with early-stage dementia, who still have moments of clarity when they are legally competent.

The supporters of a more relaxed application of euthanasia also advocate termination of the life of a person in the more advanced stages of dementia, if he had recorded earlier the stage of the disease at which his life can be terminated.

Physicians shy away from this in practice, because it is difficult to determine at which moment the life of the person with dementia should be ended. This is especially true if the demented patient whose life is about to be ended has by then forgotten he ever asked for it.

The NVVE has tried to persuade physicians to let go of this reservation. Not even disciplinary action has been ruled out as a means to coerce physicians to provide suicide or euthanasia services. The NVVE action plan quotes director Petra de Jong: "So far... only a few physicians have had the courage to provide the requested assistance to die."

In 2011, the life of a patient with advanced dementia was ended by her physician. Although the 64-year-old could not repeat her wish to die on the day she died, there was no doubt about her earlier request for euthanasia if she developed dementia. The regional euthanasia review committees found that this first case of ending the life of a patient with advanced dementia complied with the criteria.[55] It can only grow from here.

Another controversy pushed continuously by the NVVE since euthanasia became legally accepted is termination of life in children. According to the Euthanasia Act, euthanasia is permitted from the age of twelve, when children are old enough to have a say. Yet in practice termination of life also occurs in children under twelve. This is hardly surprising, as suffering does not observe age limits.

We know this thanks to a survey conducted in 2001 of medical end-of-life decisions concerning children. Physicians could report their actions anonymously, a method similar to the repeated surveys of euthanasia and termination of life without request.[56]

When the life of a child is deliberately ended, physicians generally act at the request of the parents. Yet the survey shows that there are some cases in which physicians end a child's life without a request from either the child or his parents.

---

55 Euthanasiecommissie.nl/oordelen_directory/2011/60-69_jarig_rouw_2011_123821.pdf

56 Astrid M. Vrakking, Agnes van der Heide, Willem Frans M. Arts, Rob Pieters, Edwin van der Voort, Judith A.C. Rietjens, Bregje Onwuteaka-Philipsen, Paul J. van der Maas, Gerrit van der Wal, Medical End-of-Life Decisions for Children in the Netherlands, *Arch Pediatr Adolesc Med* 2005; 159: p.802-809

Book: *In God's Chair*
A Novel About The Termination Of The Life Of An 11-Year-Old

To generate understanding for physicians who end the lives of seriously ill children, pediatrician Paul Brand published a novel in 2006, *In God's Chair* [*De stoel van God*], about the termination of the life of an 11-year-old.[57]

The author states that he has exaggerated the novel's case histories to create the drama necessary to generate debate. Apparently, this mission has been accomplished: the book has been favorably received on television and by the press.

Theo van Diepen, the young hero of the book, will never forget his grandmother's horrible deathbed, which is filled with pain in the final moments of her life.

The novel unfolds in three main "case histories." During his medical schooling Van Diepen sees an experienced colleague implicated in a scandal: he deliberately ended the life of an infant with spina bifida and hydrocephalus during a heavy epileptic seizure. To the young doctor Van Diepen, this is an example of correct medical action. By ending the child's life the colleague has avoided suffering, and that is what a physician is supposed to do: "*primum non nocere* – above all do no harm." The Public Prosecution Service made it very clear that this is not to happen again.

In the novel's second case history, the physician who is training Van Diepen takes the opposite action. Sven, a boy with a progressive muscular disease, is about to die and has great difficulty breathing.

"In an ideal world, Theo, I would now first give this boy a good shot of morphine, after consulting with his parents of course, so he can go to sleep comfortably, followed by norcuron. His muscles will become paralyzed and he will stop breathing .. and gasping. So he can drift off peacefully while his parents hold him. But the law won't let me."

That night Van Diepen says to his wife in anger: "The

---

57   Paul Brand, *De stoel van God*, Houten, Sapienta, 2006 [Sitting in God's chair]

Netherlands is the only country in the world that has every-thing legally organized, except when it comes to children."

In the third case history, Van Diepen is a specialist in pediatric lung diseases, and responsible for the treatment of Klaas, a child with cystic fibrosis. While talking with Klaas' mother Annemarie, Theo suggests "There must be some way to help children that suffer horribly to live the final days of their life in an acceptable way, no pain, no suffering, but peaceful and with dignity, and allow them a gentle death. We should be able to arrange this." "I agree with you," Annemarie replies "but that means you must to be willing to sit in God's chair. And that is not an easy chair to fill."

"No, it isn't. An easy chair. Definitely not an easy chair. But also not a chair that can be ignored. Someone has to sit in it. If you don't do anything and let the child suffer, you are still sitting in it."

As time passes, Klaas successfully contends with his disease. He becomes acquainted with Kim, a girl who shares his illness. When Kim's lung transplant fails, she first swells up beyond recognition and then she dies. Young Klaas is devastated. His parents want him to have new lungs, but he is certain that he does not want a lung transplant.

Klaas and his parents are a warm and mutually under-standing family; his parents take his refusal seriously. As Klaas deteriorates, Van Diepen again raises the theme of euthanasia. "When the moment is there, I feel I should give him something to make the dying ... more gentle, quicker... To make it right." Klaas has no objections, and neither do his parents.

Next the novel outlines the legal problems. Doctor van Diepen writes down what they discussed on paper and presents this to Klaas' parents. "When they were done reading I started to talk. About the law that forbids me to do what we had agreed on orally and on paper. Because Klaas was not yet twelve years old. The disbelief in their eyes. How could that be? If anything was unfair it must be a terminally ill child with the prospect of a horrible death. Surely the authorities, the legislator, would have to do something about it? This simply couldn't be true." Van Diepen continues: "that left me with two choices. I could attribute the death to natural causes and commit forgery. Or I could say the death was due to unnatural causes and be honest."

At age eleven, Klaas is very sick and short of breath. "I then took the syringe... Silently I looked at Klaas' face, sleeping peacefully, trusting, no pain or fear. This is how it is supposed to be, I thought... This is still my job as a physician. This is the *primum non nocere* in the Hippocratic oath I took – above all do no harm, do not cause damage. That is what I am doing now."

After Klaas' euthanasia, Theo van Diepen reports to the municipal coroner that this was not a death from natural causes. The Public Prosecutor comes forward. The courts will be involved. Theo van Diepen sighs about the lack of understanding. "Things didn't go 100% according to the regulations. But in the case of Klaas that was all so ... it just happened like this because the illness had caught up to Klaas. There was no time for legal precision grinding, for details, for laborious and extensive paperwork, for tons of red tape. A child was terminally ill and he needed to be helped. And this was the only remaining option. Which should have priority: the interest of this terminally ill child and his parents, or the law? The court would have to decide."

Then comes the verdict. "The judge looked only at the paper when she read out my sentence. Not at me." Theo van Diepen is pronounced guilty of murder, but with the observation murder is only a technical legal term in this case, and has nothing to do with what the general public understands murder to be. He receives a one-week suspended prison sentence. *In God's Chair* is a novel. It is fiction and fantasy, but the writer is unmistakably close to reality. The book provides a look into the tasks and problems, but also the thinking and actions of a physician. Moreover, physician-novelist Paul Brand is friends with Eduard Verhagen, author of the Groningen Protocol. Verhagen makes a cameo appearance in the novel. The novel poignantly describes the lives and deaths of several very ill children. Amidst the very understandable emotions in this book, the author propagates a point of view, namely that euthanasia should also be permitted in children. The way in which he attempts to convince the reader of this point of view is similar to the media examples mentioned earlier: the films, documentaries and dramas about termination of life.

In God's Chair presents the reader with an idealized image of termination of life. Family members love each other; there is no trace of animosity, arguments, conflicting interests or divorce. Harmony and mutual understanding always reign among the physician, the patient, and the parents. In the real world, are such idealized stories of any use? In addition to love and understanding the real world also contains ambition, disgust, fear, abandonment and vanity; there are non-harmonious families as well as harmonious ones.

In the novel, all natural deaths are described as gruesome. The physician's grandmother suffers unbearable pains. Sven, the second case, suffocates. Kim swells unrecognizably at the end of her life. However, when Van Diepen takes control of Klaas' dying, the deathbed is harmonious and dignified. The physician who has the guts to control the dying is portrayed as courageous.

Regulations are described in the novel as 'red tape', as 'legal precision grinding', as 'paperwork' that cannot do justice to the physician, who often has to make decisions and act under pressure of time. Whereas the people who opt for termination of life in this novel look at each other lovingly all the time, the judiciary is cold and ruthless; the judge fails to look the accused physician in the eye as she reads the verdict of murder. The judge's verdict does tie in with real life, including the observation made by the judge that what the law considers murder is not the same thing as what people actually understand the term to mean. Judges in the Netherlands do shy away from referring to termination of life that does not comply with the regulations as "murder," even when the law says it is.

In one essential aspect, *In God's Chair* contains an interesting euphemism. Hippocrates' phrase *"primum non nocere*

– above all do no harm," which every physician takes an oath to uphold, is given a whole new meaning. Theo van Diepen feels that the best way to apply this rule "above all do no harm" is by ending Klaas' life. This is new. Until now, termination of life is sometimes considered justifiable as an evil that in certain situations can be preferable to an even greater evil: suffering. But in a kind of newspeak, this novel represents termination of life by a physician as "above all do no harm."

This important point in the novel sheds light on the underlying beliefs of Van Diepen, as described by Brand. If suffering occurs, it is the physician's duty to end it. If he cannot end it by curing it, then termination of life is the next option. If the physicians of the Netherlands accepted Van Diepen's ideas, all future physicians would be instructed to avoid all suffering, if necessary by ending the lives of legally incompetent patients. Their responsibilities and power would increase in the future.

Brand's briskly selling novel has stirred up a lot of discussion, dominated by sympathetic reactions. A sixth edition has been published, more than 10,000 copies sold.

In October 2007, on Paul Brand's website *In God's Chair*, the mother of a seriously ill nine-year-old child described her worries about and her love for her son. She wondered why she is not allowed to make a case for the termination of his life. "B. has a hard life, in and out of the hospital, numerous examinations, lots of pain and sorrow, scores of associated complications … On the list of child-worthy existence his score is zero. …We grieve for B., his death won't ease our grief, but he would be free of the pain and hopelessness, the deterioration and the struggle… With all my heart I love this little man, but my grief is huge. For him, for his brother and sister, for our whole family. It is so incredibly senseless. There is no adequate place for him in an institution; they simply cannot provide this care… At home we can cherish him as much as humanly possible. …Why can't I talk about this? Why are my sentences cut short? Why is it basically taboo to express that this life is agony for every person involved? Why can you only talk about this prenatally and in the case of …competent adult patients?"[58] This mother is pleased with Paul Brand's book. She thinks that her seriously ill child would be better off if he dies.

After this reaction to Brand's novel, this mother was interviewed anonymously in the daily newspaper *NRC Handelsblad.*[59]

TELEVISION DISCUSSION: *Rondom Tien*

The Dutch public television program *Rondom Tien* picked up the discussion in 2009.[60] It gave parents of children with multiple disabilities a platform. One mother described multiple-disabled Livia (age 9): "She knows nothing, can do nothing, she really is nothing. She can pick up a toy, the same toy for the last nine years …I don't think you have children to see them suffer like this. It is pointless, and it always will be. I love her and she is my child, but I think that perhaps the ultimate expression of my love for this child is to be able to say: we can let her go, we are able let her go, it's all right, it is done, you can let go now." When asked by interviewer Cees Grimbergen whether she would consider the death of her daughter liberating, she responded "Yes." She has an agreement with her daughter's physicians that they will not treat life-threatening illnesses and she confesses she is waiting for such an illness.

In this television broadcast, Leiden ethicist Dorothea Touwen advocates speaking 'openly' with each other about multiple-disabled children, as in the earlier euthanasia discussion. What this 'openness' entails becomes clearer when Touwen says that if parents and physicians agree, foregoing treatment or active termination of life should be possible in children 'with a below minimum quality of life'. No one asks what a 'below minimum quality of life' is, or who determines it. Pediatrician Adri Burger says she asks parents whether they want treatment for their disabled child in the event it develops

---

58 www.destoelvangod.nl October 2007

59 Brigit Kooijman, "Wéér een operatie, weer pijn en verdriet," NRC Handelsblad, January 10 2009 [Another operation, More pain and grief]

60 Rondom Tien, NCRV, March 14 2009

pneumonia. Livia's mother agrees that parents should have the option of having physicians withhold treatment.

The fact that multiple-disabled children, at the request of their parents, are not always given antibiotics for pneumonia shows how making judgments about another person's life can sometimes work out in practice. The life of a child is thought to be of limited significance, which is why a simple medicine for an infection, a medication that costs little and does not hurt, is withheld.

Since the Euthanasia Act was passed, advocates have taken the battle to ever-expanding new fronts.

Chapter 5
Just One Step Further

Slippery Slope? An Inquiry

And so the situation continues to develop in the Netherlands. Every step leads one step further. We are constantly presented with new cases of people whose suffering makes us wonder whether death would be the better option for them. When euthanasia was legalized, opponents warned about the possibility of this 'slippery slope': once we accept that people can be killed by their physician at their request, soon the lives of people who do not request it will also be terminated. Eventually the value of a human life will decrease, especially when it is in less than perfect condition.

Many take hold of this 'slippery slope' concept and run with it. Both the Dutch who blindly defend everything that happens in their country, and their most severe critics abroad exaggerate this 'slippery slope'. Both groups may act as if 'slippery slope' means that accepting euthanasia on Monday means you will have Dr. Mengele sitting on your couch on Tuesday. This exaggeration is to the advantage of both groups. It allows the critics of the Netherlands to portray the Dutch euthanasia policy as Nazi-like ("Dr. Mengele is alive and he lives in Holland"), while the advocates of the Dutch approach can ridicule the concept of the 'slippery slope' ("They are calling us Nazis, how ridiculous is that?").

Exaggeration is not the intention in this book. Here the term 'slippery slope' is used to indicate that the development is entirely in one direction – each step facilitates the next one.

This seems to be the situation in the Netherlands ever since euthanasia was accepted. Initially, in the 1980s, it concerned only euthanasia in the traditional sense: a person in terrible physical pain, often as a result of cancer, in full possession of his faculties, asks a physician to end his life. In other countries that are currently considering allowing euthanasia, this classic case is invariably mentioned.

But after the Supreme Court accepted euthanasia in these classic cases, the court subsequently categorized 'mental suffering' as suffering that could be avoided by terminating life. Legally incompetent individuals, newborns, people with dementia, persons in a coma or psychiatric patients, have been the subjects of discussion since about 1990. And legal termination of life has been advocated for slightly older children who are too young to fall under the Euthanasia Act. The courts in the Netherlands have indeed accepted termination of life in severely disabled newborns after the physicians decided to discontinue medically futile treatment. Although these infants face imminent death, termination of life can sometimes be applied, if the physician judges this is the best way to avoid suffering. Subsequent to the courts' decisions, the discussion in the Netherlands expanded to include termination of life in newborns who could survive on their own, but for whom this was considered undesirable. And in 2011 the debate focused mainly on the question whether the elderly person who is not ill but is tired of life has the right to request assistance to end his life.

From the classic understanding of euthanasia to termination of life in disabled newborns whose survival is considered undesirable, is unmistakably a considerable development. The road from assisted suicide because a person is in pain as a result of cancer, to assisted suicide because a person is old and weary of life is also quite impressive.

You may be of the opinion that the shift in the Netherlands' position is disgraceful. Or perhaps you are of the opinion that in all of these cases termination of life is sometimes the best of the available options. The one thing you cannot do is deny that the boundaries have been continually pushed back, moving the Netherlands a considerable distance from its original position. The discussion about one category of people for whom termination of life is accepted draws attention to an adjacent category of individuals to whom the same arguments for termination of life can be applied. And so the position of the Netherlands is constantly shifting. Again, we need not consider this a disgrace. Yet the shift itself cannot be denied.

If we continue on this road, we may open the discussion to termination of the lives of legally incompetent disabled adolescents or adults, if the people around them feel that they are suffering hopelessly. Ethicist and liberal (VVD) politician Heleen Dupuis advocated this years ago. In her opinion we should consider termination of the lives of patients who are saved by a medical intervention "as soon as the results are disappointing."[61] Incidentally, she considers warnings about the slippery slope "disgraceful."[62]

This is not an unusual pattern: the most vociferous advocates of expanding the scope of termination of life are also the ones who get the angriest at those who suggest that the slippery slope does exist. Euthanasia association NVVE is sick and tired of the slippery-slope warning. In the book entitled *Euthanasia, The Practice From a Different Perspective*[*Euthanasie, de praktijk anders bekeken*], Jacob Kohnstamm, then president of the NVVE and former politician for left-wing liberal party D66, wrote that there is no gradual shift. "Slippery slope? Again, there simply is no such thing." Yet in the same preface he makes a case for allowing euthanasia for reasons of 'suffering from life' for elderly people mentioned before. Such assisted suicide is currently not allowed

---

61 Heleen M. Dupuis, Wel of niet behandelen? Baat het niet, dan schaadt het wél, Baarn, Ambo, 1994 [Treat or not treat? It does hurt to try]

62 Dupuis, H.M., Mag er nog gestorven worden? Het toenemende imperatief van de technologie, in: Boon, Leo (red), *Beslissen over leven en dood. Dilemmabij wilsonbekwame ernstig-gehandicapte pasgeborenen, coma-patiënten, zwakzinnigen en psycho-geriatrische patiënten*, Amstelveen, Sympoz, 1989 [Are we allowed to die anymore? Technology's increasing imperative]

in law, and it would require an extension of the group of people for whom termination of life is possible. That, too, is the next step forward (or back). This next step invariably happens: one form of termination of life results in a call for the next.

To illustrate: four days after Dutch Minister of Public Health Els Borst successfully guided the Euthanasia Act through parliament, she gave an interview in which she advocated legalizing assisted suicide for people who are tired of life. "I have seen a person in this situation up close and later I talked to another. Both were 95 years old and both were simply fed up. They were bored out of their minds and unfortunately they were not bored to death."[63] Legalizing one type of termination of life immediately draws attention to the next category of people for whom voluntary euthanasia is not allowed, but suddenly appears to make sense.

Is the Netherlands really slipping? Yes, says British legal scholar John Keown, it is unmistakably slipping in the wrong direction since the Supreme Court permitted euthanasia. He presents as evidence the approximately one thousand cases a year in which the lives of people who did not ask for it are terminated, as was made public in 1991.[64]

But in the Netherlands' universities, the young generation of Dutch students are being taught "No, there is no slippery slope." In the authoritative *Dutch Health Law Handbook*, experts Gevers and Legemaate swiftly put an end to the fear of a slippery slope. "…in exceptional cases termination of life without request cannot be avoided, but the assumption that, by allowing euthanasia, society will accept termination of life without request as normal is unfounded." Note: their only argument is that "in exceptional cases termination of life without request cannot be avoided." This tends to confirm the existence of a slippery slope. Gevers and Legemaate continue: "Even experience does not support the risk of

---

63   "Ik kan me goed voorstellen dat artsen stervenshulp niet melden." Minister Borst over het tekort van de nieuwe euthanasiewet, NRC Handelsblad, April 14 2001 ["I understand why physicians do not report assisted dying" Minister Els Borst on the shortcoming of the new Euthanasia Act; April 14 2001]

64   Keown, op. cit., p. 115 ff

slipping, as the results of the fourth empirical study into medical end-of-life decisions from 2007 illustrates."[65] However, this study shows – yet again - that in the Netherlands lives are terminated without request hundreds of times a year. And this, goes the international argument, proves the existence of the slippery slope. Instead of refuting the criticism, this handbook, without presenting a single argument, claims: there is no slippery slope in the Netherlands.

American-Dutch scholar John Griffiths has spoken out in defense of the Netherlands. You have not proven a slippery slope, he said, unless you can prove that more people who did not ask for it are killed in the Netherlands than in other countries.[66] Foreign observers, shocked by the Dutch figures showing that people are regularly killed without request, use the numbers to substantiate their criticism of the Dutch policy. However, Griffiths argues, other countries do not conduct research of a similar scale and precision into physicians and their patients' end of life. Therefore, says Griffiths, it is impossible for critics to claim that the situation in the Netherlands is worse than anywhere else.

Another way to demonstrate a slippery slope, according to Griffiths, is to establish that there has been an increase of non-voluntary euthanasia in the Netherlands since euthanasia has been allowed, as compared to before the court decisions. This is also impossible, because – again – no figures are available. Surveys of termination of life in the Netherlands did not start until 1990. Perhaps the current situation in the Netherlands is much better than before, or better than other countries. Perhaps, Griffiths argues, the Dutch openness is a way to prevent sliding down the slippery slope.

Griffiths' argument is just as easily turned around. Dutch experts can be very quick to suggest that what is studied and discussed openly in

---

65 Leenen, H.J.J., J.K.M. Gevers, J. Legemaate, *Handboek gezondsheidsrecht. Deel 1. Rechten van mensen in de gezondheidszorg*, Houten, Bohn Stafleu van Loghum, 2007, vijfde geheel herziene druk, p. 341 [Dutch Health Law Handbook. Part 1. Rights of persons in healthcare]

66 John Griffiths, Heleen Weyers, Maurice Adams, *Euthanasia and Law in Europe*, Oxford and Portland, Oregon, Hart Publishing, 2008, p. 513

the Netherlands must be happening on the sly elsewhere, and that there-fore everything is much worse abroad. Yet like their opponents, these defenders of the Netherlands have no figures to base their assertions on; for they have no proof that physicians are secretly terminating lives abroad, let alone the scale on which it happens. Figures are only avail-able for the Netherlands, making comparison impossible. This once again demonstrates that the repeated survey of life-terminating action, undertaken by physicians in the Netherlands since 1990, is unparalleled.

When in 2003 the British House of Lords debated the issue of life-shortening action by physicians, Griffiths stood up for the heavi-ly-criticized Netherlands. The British were afraid that if you legalized euthanasia you would soon also legalize non-voluntary termination of life. Nonsense, said Griffiths: "It is certainly possible to allow the first and forbid the second."[67] Griffiths was honest enough to admit that the Netherlands did in fact allow first one and then the other in the courts. First came euthanasia, then termination of life without request, and both times the courts permitted it because it ended hopeless and unbearable suffering. However, this sequence was not necessary, Griffiths contend-ed. The courts could have permitted euthanasia, but not gone on to ac-cept termination of life without request. So – says Griffiths – there is no slippery slope.

There is a flaw in his reasoning. Griffiths disregards the demonstrat-ed fact that arguments used in favor of those classic cases of self-deter-mined euthanasia can also be used in cases far outside those limits. It will be tempting to continually take it one step further. Once you accept that sometimes it is allowed to avoid suffering by killing a person, it won't be easy to find a new boundary.

In everyday life you can hear this happening. Sometimes people say that "for me personally, if I can't do that anymore, I don't want to go on." This concerns them personally and making your own decisions is within the boundaries of the Dutch Euthanasia Act. Yet it is only natural

---

67 John Griffiths, Dutch Data in the International Debate: A Statement by John Griffiths at a Briefing Session at the House of Lords, *MBPSL Newsletter* October 2003, No. 8

to use the same argument for another person: "John has been in a coma for years, you wouldn't want that for yourself, would you? I think we should allow him to die with dignity."

The underlying argument in all of this is that it is better to end hopeless and unbearable suffering by ending the life of the person who suffers. It is almost impossible to confine this argument to the realm of self-determination. As soon as you accept suffering as a basis for euthanasia, you can insist upon the equality of legally competent and incompetent people to require that you also end, without request, their 'hopeless and unbearable suffering': "Surely you don't want to let a person suffer simply because he is mentally disabled and unable to ask for euthanasia?" The argument in favor of euthanasia is then logically applied to an incompetent person.

The result, however, is that an argument from the realm of self-determination is used to justify the ultimate opposite of self-determination: killing someone who can't fight back.

How Strict Are The 'Strict Criteria Of Due Care'?

To prevent slipping on a slippery slope you could try to dig your heels in. So even if there already was a slippery slope, you would not automatically slide all the way down. You slide down only as far as you want. You can draw a line, can't you? Obviously the risk of a slippery slope would diminish considerably, and perhaps even disappear, if conditions were attached to termination of life.

All types of termination of life in the Netherlands are subject to 'due care' conditions that are invariably characterized by supporters as "strict" or "very strict." In real life, however, the due care criteria are sometimes relaxed, disregarded or brushed aside, by the same people who emphasize the safety of the care exercised by Dutch physicians.

Winnie Sorgdrager, former politician of left-wing liberal party D66 and until recently chair of a committee that reviews reported cases of euthanasia, has proven flexible when it comes to applying the rules. In an article in the reputable newspaper *Trouw* she wrote about the sneaking doubt she sometimes feels when she sees the resolute signatures of patients at the bottom of euthanasia requests, while they were so sick they could barely hold a pen. "Sometimes there are very robust signatures from persons who are dying and that quickly leads to the question "Who did the signing?" The committees are not criminal investigation departments, but the fact that we are more or less convinced that another person signed the request does not feel right."[68]

So what would Sorgdrager do? Would she forward this case to the Public Prosecution Service? No, because the request for euthanasia does not need to be signed on paper – it can also be made orally. For this reason Sorgdrager wrote that she was not too upset when she was confronted with a signed euthanasia request with a suspected forged signature.

In the article, Sorgdrager wrote that even when her review committee suspected that the signature on the bottom of the form was probably forged, the committee still decided to give the green light to the euthanasia. Such decisions were never presented to the Public Prosecution Service, so the courts were never able to evaluate them. This concerns an important legal precondition for euthanasia: the question whether the life was really terminated at the request of the patient him/herself.

Sorgdrager is a former Minister of Justice. The amazing thing is that she actually wrote this article, which recounted how flexible her review committee was regarding suspected forged signatures, to extol the excellent way in which the Dutch deal with this difficult subject.

Sorgdrager's actions did not go unchallenged. Ethicist Theo Boer was of the three members of the review committee headed by Winnie Sorgdrager. In an interview in 2008, he shared that, in view of the doubts whether the papers were signed by the patient, he would have preferred to refer these cases to the PPS. The majority of the committee decided differently. One of the deciding factors was that the euthanasia

---

68   Winnie Sorgdrager, "De arts, de jurist, de ethicus en de dood," *newspaper Trouw*, January 5 2008, Letter & Geest p. 1-3 [The physician, the lawyer, the ethicist and death]

law does not formally require an advance directive. Another was that the few times the committee inquired about the origin of the signature, the physicians involved all confirmed that it really was the patient's signature. As the review committees have no investigative powers, it was decided to let the physician's word be the deciding factor.[69] No judge was ever involved in any of these cases.

Even the cases that do make it to the courts are generally treated leniently in the Netherlands. In 1997 Amsterdam physician Van Oijen ended the life of a patient, a dying woman. The woman did not ask him to do this. However, it was a difficult death, and the woman's daughters asked the doctor to end their mother's suffering.

It is not uncommon for families to make such a request. During the evaluation of the Euthanasia Act in 2005, the researchers determined that physicians mention a "request or wish of family" as one of the "main reasons to perform euthanasia or assisted suicide" in eleven percent of all euthanasia cases.[70] This contradicts the words of the Euthanasia Act, which declares that a request from a relative would have no influence.

But some physicians definitely listen to family, as Dr. Van Oijen did when the daughters of the dying patient requested that he terminate her life. He just happened to have with him a potentially lethal medication – past its expiration date by the way – and immediately administered it. He subsequently wrote on the death certificate that she had died a "natural death." This termination of life most certainly did not meet the due care criteria. The woman did not die at her own request and the physician signed a false death certificate. The court sentenced Dr. Van Oijen to a suspended fine for lying about the cause of death. While the court spoke of punishable "murder," it did not impose punishment for the termination of life. In fact, it immediately added that it did not really resemble murder. On the contrary, the court held that Van Oijen acted in good conscience.

---

69   Interview with Theo Boer, February 19 2008

70   Onwuteaka, op. cit., p. 104

On appeal the court was slightly sterner: it imposed a suspended custodial sentence for murder, but also added some remarks to the effect that it was not really murder. Furthermore the appeal court said that the simple fact that the woman did not request euthanasia herself was not enough reason to call it murder. More than anything, the court was bothered by the fact that the physician lied about it. Finally, the highest judge, the Supreme Court, confirmed the ruling.

Although this physician violated almost every aspect of the law, after this verdict he was portrayed by many people in the Netherlands as a martyr.

The physician Ben Crul is a staunch proponent of the Dutch euthanasia practice. He has defended its voluntary nature on French television. Crul hastened to justify Van Oijen's act of non-voluntary termination of life. According to Crul, who is also editor-in-chief of the medical journal *Medisch Contact*, this is not murder, but rather "assisted dying." The *Dutch Right-to-Die Association* NVVE, the organization that for years had publicly emphasized the voluntary nature of euthanasia, also spoke out in defense of Dr. Van Oijen, who had trampled on almost every due care requirement for euthanasia. Criminal law is "too static" for such complex real-life cases, the NVVE declared, thereby indicating that the "strict" conditions for euthanasia can be brushed aside in real life. The *Royal Dutch Medical Association* KNMG also spoke up for their colleague. They stated that Van Oijen, who was convicted of murder, had acted "with integrity." The KNMG further suggested that these cases of non-voluntary termination of life should be taken out of the courts to be assessed by regional review committees.

Perhaps Van Oijen had so many defenders because this doctor was popular in the Dutch euthanasia movement. He was featured in the first documentary to portray euthanasia, the 1994 Dutch television documentary *Death on Request* [*Dood op verzoek*] which was also broadcast in other countries.

Apparently, a physician can totally ignore the "strict requirements" that apply to euthanasia and still enjoy the trust of the legal-medical establishment in the Netherlands. The alarm bells that should go off when physicians engage in illegal termination of life are not working. While the courts spoke sternly of "murder," they only imposed suspended sentences, and hastened to say that this was not really murder. Even today, defenders stand up who feel that the courts were much too hard on Van Oijen.

If they criticized the physicians who do not meet the "strict requirements," it would benefit the credibility of euthanasia advocates. They don't. The euthanasia movement actually defends these physicians. The boundaries are not guarded; on the contrary, they are pushed back. One thing evidently does lead to another, confirming that there is indeed a slippery slope.

The Arguments That Brought Us Here

How did we reach this point that under certain circumstances it is allowed to judge that another person is better off dead and to act on that judgment? An overview of the arguments that brought us here:

1. The Argument Of Advancing Technology

"Would you prefer that people are kept alive hooked up to machines and with tubes sticking out everywhere?"

This is the classic argument of the euthanasia movement. The reasoning is that medical technology advances so rapidly that we are forced to make choices the generations before us did not have to make. Physicians are able to prolong life much more frequently than before, but is this always what we want? Should we do everything simply because we can?

The argument seems ironclad, but isn't. It is only ironclad when you pretend there are only two options: saving the life, or active termination of life by the physician. In reality there is a third option: foregoing medical options, but also foregoing termination of life, and so opting for a natural death.

2. The Argument Of The Shocking Example

"Immediately after birth it becomes clear that the baby has a very serious skin disease. His daily care and changing the dressing are extremely painful"

The strongest argument for termination of life without request is the existence of horrifying conditions. Sometimes these affect people that are unable to make their own decisions, like newborns. Situations of necessity happen. They are not fiction.

Describing a problem by means of a concrete case is compelling in any debate, because these are concrete people in concrete situations. Yet this is no reason to stop the debate about the main issues. We must continue to ask the question whether the newborn in this example would be better off dead and if so, whether this is reason to kill him.

3. The "Dead Is Dead" Argument

"If you feel that there are situations in which it is better to discontinue a person's treatment and you know the effect will be that he dies, then you might as well go for termination of life, because the outcome is the same in both cases"

Many people accept that there are situations in which it is better to forego medical treatment, even if this results in the death of the patient. The people who accept this are often asked why they are against termination of life, as the outcome is the same. Dead is dead. Protestant theologian Harry Kuitert successfully used this argument in the Netherlands to remove resistance, first against termination of life with request, and later without request.

It is a weak argument. In one situation the person dies of a disease, and in the other situation because the physician acts to end his life. The outcome may be the same, but the methods are not. The argument is also weak because it presumes that if the end serves a moral purpose, then the means are always morally justified. It is about the goal. The goal determines whether the methods are ethically sound. The end justifies the means.

This is diametrically opposed to the concept of human rights. Human beings, regardless of what happens, have certain rights that no one can take away from them. No matter how wonderful the goal, if it can only be reached by violating a human right, then it should not be pursued. Letting die and causing to die are therefore not morally equal.

4. The Argument Of The "Medical End-Of-Life Decisions"

"The decision not to treat a person is a more fundamental decision than the potential subsequent decision to end his life"

Related to argument three is the reasoning that we can avoid asking ourselves whether termination of life is permissible, either with or without request, if there has been a previous decision to withdraw treatment. The decision to end a person's life does not really matter; the preceding decision to not provide medical treatment to a person is much more important. At that point the decision is made that treatment would be hopeless or pointless and the approaching death must be accepted.

This argument is a diversionary action. Whether ending a person's life can be morally justified is only one part of the larger complex of difficult questions that must be answered just before the end of life. Although the question must be asked, this does not erase the difference between causing to die and letting die.

5. The Activism Argument

"We must do something, doing nothing is not an option"

Sometimes we face difficult dilemmas and require us to do something, according to the supporters of termination of life. Sometimes we must choose the least bad option.

This argument is one that politicians like to use in all kinds of completely different discussions. The argument's great weakness is that it does not answer the obvious question: why? Why is doing nothing not an option?

We could also act to take the best possible care of a person until his death occurs naturally. The activism argument pretends that people don't die if they are not helped to die. This is obviously less than accurate. Not acting, or doing nothing, is definitely an option.

A further problem is that the activism argument expands the physician's job: if the physician is unable to prevent his patient suffering, he is obligated to make sure the patient dies.

6. The Courage Argument

"We must have the guts to face up to the fact that sometimes it is better for a person to die, and if death is long in coming, a physician must have the courage to bring it closer."

According to this argument, it is cowardly to hide behind the 'taboo' that a physician should not kill. A courageous physician can sometimes decide, out of compassion, to cause a person to die. Imagine that a decision has been made to discontinue treatment of a newborn. The death of the child therefore becomes inevitable. This argument states it is cowardly to wait until death occurs naturally, and courageous to administer death immediately.[71]

Contradicting this argument is the fact that this adds new obligations to the role of the physician. Foregoing medical treatment means that the patient can die when that time comes. He then dies of the untreated disease. According to the courage argument, the physician should have the courage to bring the moment of death forward by killing the patient. The implicit suggestion is that a physician who waits for his patient to die a natural death is a coward.

This argument is often used in combination with the dead-is-dead argument and the activism argument.

---

71   For an example of this argument see reasoning of physician and lecturer on medical ethics S. van de Vathorst, De dood als beste optie. Levensbeëindiging van een pasgeborene is soms morele plicht, in: Medisch Contact 58, 2003, p. 1471-173 [Death as the best option. Termination of life in newborns is sometimes a moral duty]

7. The Inevitability Argument

"It will inevitably happen, let's discuss the conditions un-
der which it is allowed so we can at least control it"

This line of reasoning is widely used in the Netherlands. Consider the nursing home physician who wrote in 1989: "terminating the life of chronic coma patients is inevitable."[72] Since it is inevitable, we should therefore prepare ourselves for it.

Instead of debating whether the new practice is indeed inevitable, the discussion is confined to the conditions under which the inevitable is allowed to happen. As soon as rules and conditions are formulated, however, there is no way back. The 'inevitable' becomes an entrenched reality.

This argument does not hold water because it doesn't answer the question *why*. Why is termination of life in chronic coma patients inevitable?

8. The Argument Of Openness

"At least the Netherlands is open and honest, in other
countries they do it on the sly"

One very popular argument is that here in the Netherlands, we do openly what other countries do surreptitiously. We, the Dutch, are honest and sincere; we 'break taboos' by making them subjects of discussion, which at the very least makes what is happening anyway transparent and controllable. Abroad, on the other hand, they 'enforce taboos' on termination of life. This forces physicians to do it on the sly, so there is no control.

The weakness of this argument is that it cannot be proven. There are no figures to compare situations. To simply assume that what happens

---

72   Bakker-Winnubst in: Boon, Leo (red.), Beslissen over leven en dood. Dilemmas bij
      wilsonbekwame ernstig-gehandicapte pasgeborenen, coma-patiënten, zwakzinnigen en
      psycho-geriatrische patiënten, Amstelveen, Sympoz, 1989, p. 76 [Life-and-death decisions.
      Dilemmas in incompetent, severely disabled newborns, coma patients, mentally retarded
      and psychogeriatric patients]

openly in the Netherlands must be happening secretly in other countries is jumping to conclusions. The reverse argument is just as easy to make: the chance that people are being killed without request is larger in a country that allows euthanasia than in countries reluctant to practice medical killing. There is no proof for either claim.

9. The Equality Argument

"If people who are of sound mind are allowed to opt for voluntary euthanasia, it is a question of equality to also put legally incompetent individuals who suffer hopelessly and unbearably out of their misery."

As long as their goal was to make voluntary termination of life acceptable, the euthanasia movement vehemently denied this argument. It was very quick to use this extremely logical argument later: if a legally competent individual who suffers hopelessly and unbearably can request euthanasia, then we can also end the life of a severely suffering child, or person with Alzheimer's disease or a mental disability.

This argument is incompatible with the principle of patient self-determination, which is central to the *public* euthanasia debate. In this argument, we decide for another person that it is better for him to die.

If we assume that euthanasia is less about self-determination, and more about pity, this argument gains strength. In that case we can view termination of life as an option to avoid suffering in legally incompetent individuals. Termination of life thus becomes a form of 'mercy killing'. This is patronizing, the very opposite of self-determination. The euthanasia movement that always insisted that the autonomous patient is central, is actually advocating categorically opposite arguments at the same time.

10. The Trust Argument 1

"Dutch physicians wouldn't do such a thing"

The dangers outlined by the opponents of termination of life might apply to the situation in other countries, but do not apply in the

Netherlands. Physicians here, the supporters of the practice of termination of life without request claim, are extremely careful when dealing with this subject matter.

You cannot base the rule of law on this argument. All law, any law, is intended for those cases in which things do not automatically go well, cases in which people *do* violate each other's trust.

Undoubtedly the vast majority of Dutch physicians are completely trustworthy. That is not enough reason to assume that all are.

11. The Trust Argument 2

"Parents definitely don't make such a decision lightly"

When parents agree to have the life of their severely disabled newborn or child terminated, they are obviously in a very difficult situation. So difficult that, according to this argument, outsiders should respect any decision the parents make under these circumstances, regardless of the outcome.

The parents of the severely disabled child apparently enjoy a great deal of trust. So much so, that they are even trusted when they decide to have the physician end the life of their child. How this relates to the rights of the child is not discussed. Whereas in all other situations of care parents must consider child welfare, this is not considered relevant in the case of termination of life for reasons of illness or disabilities.

Without a doubt the vast majority of parents will strive to do what is best for their child in good faith. Yet here again, this is not enough reason to simply assume they do. Once again, the rule of law cannot be built on trust alone. Moreover, people may fall into a personal crisis when they learn that a person they feel responsible for is severely disabled. This can render decision-making difficult. This problem is all the more pressing if the parents' decision affects the life of their child.

12. The Argument Of The Law

"You don't understand. Termination of life without request is forbidden and prosecuted in the Netherlands. It only happens incidentally in extreme situations of necessity, but then we are really talking about very rare cases"

It is not allowed. It rarely happens. It can always be prosecuted as murder. Supporters of the flexible line emphasize that termination of life without request is not allowed in law, and happens only in the rarest of situations.

This is not a strong argument, for three reasons. First: no one checks whether termination of life without request really is rare, or that it occurs only in situations of necessity. Many cases of termination of life without request are not reported. If they are reported, which has happened especially in the case of newborns, they are rarely prosecuted by the Public Prosecution Service.

Second: although the law prohibits termination of life without request, we do not apply this law consistently in the Netherlands. The argument that the law prohibits it is therefore reminiscent of Dutch politicians who reassuringly inform other countries that soft drugs are forbidden in the Netherlands, which is true according to the letter of the law, but is not true in real life.

Third: people who shoot holes in a law and subsequently hide behind the same law are not very convincing.

13. The Argument Of Due Care

"We only do it under strict conditions"

To persuade critics of the Dutch practice we ensure them that we work very carefully in the Netherlands. It's not like we improvise. We have protocols, and strict 'due care' requirements.

The problem is that the due care requirements are merely procedural. Procedures are no answer to questions of principle. Foreign critics in particular feel that the Dutch procedures, no matter how careful, do not provide an answer to the fundamental question of what legitimizes killing people without their request. The answer to the question what about the right to life of a severely disabled newborn or an elderly person with dementia simply cannot be provided on the basis of a procedure, like checking off boxes on a form. You can demand that one, two, or ten physicians, and one, two, or all relatives agree, you can set up expert committees to approve the case either before or after the fact. The question how termination of life without request is to be reconciled with the human right that guarantees every person protection of life, cannot be answered in this way. The fundamental discussion in the Netherlands never crystallized, because we moved on to procedures right away.

In addition, we have already noted that the courts have judged violations of the due care requirements very leniently.

14. The Incomparability Argument

"Each case is different, you cannot regulate this"

It goes without saying that every life is different. The termination-of-life discussion emerges in very different circumstances. Anyone asking for general rules and principles is viewed as rigid, as someone who disregards the uniqueness of the individuals involved.

The rule of law would be utterly destroyed by this argument. The rule of law is an attempt to use generally applicable guidelines in a variety of concrete cases.

This argument is furthermore insincere. Those who plead that each case for termination of life is different, apply the same general rule always and everywhere: some life is so sad that it is better to end it.

15. The Argument Of Defining Away

"It's not about that at all"

An attack on the Dutch practice can often be countered by sidelining it. You simply say that the attacker is talking about a different subject.

In the 1980s this was done by narrowing the definition of 'euthanasia' in Dutch to mean active termination of life on request, whereas 'euthanasia' in other countries generally comprises all types of termination of life by a physician. Critics predicting that the Dutch acceptance of euthanasia would lead to termination of life without request for reasons of pity, could be dismissed by countering that such a thing was not euthanasia. We now know the critics were right to sound the alarm: in addition to 'euthanasia' in the Dutch sense (i.e. voluntary euthanasia), we now also have termination of life without request. Although the latter is no longer part of the Dutch definition, it certainly is part of Dutch reality.

The same is happening with regard to termination of life in newborns. Some physicians feel there is no termination of life when the physician kills the newborn after the decision to forego treatment, and death is near. In their definition, termination of life only concerns a newborn who could survive on its own, but whose survival is undesirable due to current or future suffering. In fact, there are many cases each year in which futile medical treatment is withdrawn from newborns. According to this extremely narrow definition of termination of life, administering a lethal dose of drugs is 'normal medical practice'.

The weakness of the argument is that it uses a quarrel about language to change the debate, but that quarrel does not change reality.

16. The Argument Of The Plural Society

"Thankfully we no longer live in a time when the government or the church can tell us what to do. In a plural society people must be able to decide for themselves"

This argument originates in the 1980s and '90s, a period when all debate on societal values and standards was avoided in the Netherlands. Instead, the individual's right to lead his life as he saw fit trumped all.

But don't we need the state, especially in a plural society where everyone else can shout out their opinion in the loudest voice, to protect the weakest members who have no voice?

If the question is whether it is allowed to end another person's life 'for his own good' we also run up against the boundaries of liberalism and self-determination. Is the family allowed to decide that someone is better off dead? Is that not contrary to this patient's right to self-determination?

17. The Post-Christian Argument

"I assume you are saying this based on your Christian beliefs. I respect that, but I am not a Christian and I expect you to respect my beliefs too"

People who express doubt or resistance to termination of life are often assumed to do this based on religious considerations. As a considerable part of the Dutch population no longer adheres to the Christian faith, they conclude that it is not necessary to listen to these Christian objections.

This line of reasoning would make sense if Christians brandishing passages from the Bible were trying to convince non-Christians. However, if Christians who object to termination of life use only arguments that are not rooted in their faith, non-Christians should have no problem listening to them. Human rights, for example, often have an unmistakable Christian essence for Christians, but are also valued by non-Christians. If a Christian refers to human rights in the debate, non-Christians should take them seriously. Yet they often don't, suggesting with a single reference to the Christian faith that they do not have to listen to him because he is a member of a minority that, although respectable, does not warrant being taken seriously. Indeed, there are examples of non-Christians who, after objecting to forms of termination of life, are assumed to be Christians and thus placed outside the debate.[73]

What this argument basically says is that we do not have to debate each other if we believe different things. This is an unusual interpretation of 'debate'.

---

73   Raphael Cohen-Almagor p. 129, p. 149

Finally, this argument does not recognize the many Protestant Christians in the Netherlands who have argued in favor of legalizing euthanasia.

18. The Short-Life Expectancy Argument

"A baby has a very short time to live, terminating its life only shortens the suffering"

This argument is presented by, among others, the ethical committees of the Dutch Pediatric Association NVK when they plead for termination of life in severely afflicted newborns.[74]

The weakness of this argument is that it is the exact opposite of the following argument.

19. The Long-Life Expectancy Argument

"A disabled newborn will live a long time and will therefore suffer for a long time. Termination of life will prevent this suffering"

Some physicians have used this argument as justification for terminating the lives of severely disabled newborns. They claim that the suffering increases the longer a disabled person lives.[75]

The amazing thing is that the ethical committee of the Dutch Pediatric Association NVK on one and the same page in a 2007 article uses both the long life expectancy and the opposite short life expectancy as potential reasons for termination of life. This creates the impression that a position is taken first: the baby is better off dead. Arguments are found afterwards.

---

[74] A.A.E. Verhagen, M.A.H.B.M. van der Hoeven, J.B. van Goudoever, M.C. de Vries, A.Y.N. Schouten-van Meeteren, M.J.I.J. Alberts, Uitzichtloos en ondraaglijk lijden en actieve levensbeëindiging bij pasgeborenen, *Nederlands Tijdschrift voor Geneeskunde* 2007; 151: p. 1474-1477 [Hopeless and unbearable suffering and active termination of life in newborns]

[75] The authors of the Groningen Protocol for termination of life in newborns use this argument, f.e. in their article A.A.E. Verhagen, J.J. Sol, O.F. Brouwer, P.J. Sauer, Actieve levensbeëindiging bij pasgeborenen in Nederland; analyse van alle 22 meldingen uit 1997/'04, *Nederlands Tijdschrift voor Geneeskunde* 2005; 149: 183-188 [Active termination of life in newborns in the Netherlands; analysis of all 22 reported cases 1997/2004]

20. The Education Argument

"The experts have pondered this exceedingly complex and difficult subject with great care for many years. Some people react very strongly now because they don't understand and they think that we are just improvising here in the Netherlands. We are doing nothing of the kind, but we understand the response, because it is all very emotional. That is why we are now going to educate the public"

This argument is used especially against the foreign critics of the Dutch practice of termination of life, but even Dutch critics are sometimes labeled as ignorant. The assumption is that "our critics just don't know enough about the subject. We experts can understand their confusion, because these are very complex problems. They need education by experts."

In reality the Dutch practice of termination of life is not that complex: the goal is to avoid suffering, and termination of life is one way to accomplish it. National and international critics have no problem understanding that concept. They don't agree with it.

Besides, this is actually a technocratic argument: the experts tell people who have a different opinion to hold their tongues. Yield to what the better-informed experts have to say. The experts assume that the criticism is the result of a lack of knowledge. If the critics only knew more about the subject, say the technocrats, they would undoubtedly agree with the experts.

21. To Declare Outrageous

"Suggesting this is an outrageous accusation; in the Netherlands we deal with this subject matter with the utmost care"

Sometimes the criticized party plays the emotional card and becomes enraged. International criticism in particular is often declared outrageous and disposed of in this way.

The weakness of simply declaring criticism 'outrageous' is that it does not address the arguments. It is only a limited display of emotions.

22. The "Foreigners-Are-Crazy" Argument

"An American tourist who broke her leg in Amsterdam resisted being treated in a Dutch hospital screaming hysterically, because she was afraid she would be euthanized."76

International criticism is sometimes ridiculed by exaggerating it. Of course criticism from other countries on the Dutch practice of termination of life is sometimes based on 'facts' that are indisputably not the case. Referring to those 'incorrect facts', however, is not enough to deal with all international criticism. Some international critics are very well informed and ask questions to which we in the Netherlands do not always have answers. However, it is indefensible to pick up only the exaggerated criticism from other countries, and then repeat them with exaggerated frequency, in the hope that this will make all criticism sound ridiculous.

---

76 The example is taken from Paul Brand, *De stoel van God* [Sitting in God's chair], Maarn, Sapienta, 2005, p. 163

Chapter 6

Self-Determination Or Compassion?

An Influential Little Book: *Medical power and medical ethics*

In the Netherlands today, you are permitted to choose your own death if you experience hopeless and unbearable suffering. Many locate the most important reason for such voluntary euthanasia in self-determination: the person who is suffering can determine to die.

However, there has been tension between compassion (or pity) and self-determination in the thirty years leading up to the Dutch Euthanasia Act of 2001. While many people feel that the emphasis is on self-determination, initially the supporters of euthanasia were more interested in mercy or compassion, in deciding for another person. The euthanasia debate started around 1969 around the idea that suffering people are sometimes better off dead, and physicians should act accordingly.

In that year, physician and scientist Jan Hendrik van den Berg started the Netherlands thinking about the sense and nonsense of medical action. His book *Medical Power And Medical Ethics* [*Medische macht en medische ethiek*], published in 1969, heavily influenced the Dutch debate. Twenty editions of the booklet were printed over a period of seven years. The Netherlands, unlike other Western countries, had avoided all discussion about euthanasia up to that point. After this book appeared, the Dutch took the lead position in the worldwide discussion about the subject.

According to Van den Berg's criticism, physicians must stop treating patients at any cost. Technology must be put in its place. Sometimes death is better than a life hooked up to machines.

People who considered themselves progressive and open-minded have quoted Van den Berg and made euthanasia a subject for discussion ever since. Long after this thin but influential booklet appeared in 1969, experts still express their appreciation for the man who initiated the euthanasia debate in the Netherlands. "The plea for a new medical ethic by Van den Berg in the 1960s can be identified as the starting point" wrote the *Commission for the Acceptability of Life Terminating Action* (CAL) of the *Royal Dutch Medical Association* KNMG in 1997[77]. "The author forces the reader to cross the boundary into the unpleasant to clarify that medical action has positive intentions, and can also have major negative consequences."

So what is it in this little book that has made 'termination of life' such a subject of discussion in the Netherlands? How does Van den Berg create a moral space to formulate a "new code of medical ethics" that would leave more room for letting, and if necessary, causing to die?

Medical Power And Medical Ethics is written in the style of a pamphlet. It describes several examples of severely disabled individuals, presented by Van den Berg as proof of unacceptable medical action. They should not be here, wrote Van den Berg, and we must blame the physicians that they are. Some of the disabled persons in the book were completely incompetent. Others were of sound mind, and therefore competent. Van den Berg did not let any of them speak.

Thalidomide babies were often in the news in the 1960s. These children were born with malformations of the limbs and other disorders, because their mothers used the drug Thalidomide during pregnancy. In 1969 Van den Berg was very outspoken about these babies: "There

---

77   R.J.M. Dillmann (et al.), *Medisch handelen rond het levenseinde bij wilsonbekwame patiënten*, Commissie Aanvaardbaarheid Levensbeëindigend handelen KNMG, Houten/ Diegem, Bohn Stafleu Van Logchum, 1997, p. 9 [Medical practice around the end of life of incompetent patients]

were parents who did not want to see their Thalidomide baby and rejected it. That seems to me a natural reaction. There were parents who, after much deliberation, killed their Thalidomide baby. That seems to me an act of courage and of dignity. There have been physicians who, following a plea from the parents, administered a fatal injection to the Thalidomide babies shortly after birth. This appears to me to be an act of simple, medical duty."

"I must assume that these lines are also read by parents who spared a severely damaged child, and who may even at this moment be watching it wandering through their home with their prostheses. …I want to ask these parents to reserve judgment for a moment. Have they not considered the question whether what they did was right? Looking at their child, did misery not seize them by the throat more than once? … My words must have been their words. They learned to steel themselves against those words, to the degree that nothing shows anymore. Consistent with this attitude they learned to treat their child with extra love, perhaps making it the center of the family. Everything can be sacrificed to the deformed child; the parents' desires, as well as the desires, and even the needs of the other children in the family. I have no kind words for that. I have no appreciation for parents whose severely deformed child no longer throws them into a panic. If my words break down their armor then they have found their mark."[78]

But Van den Berg named more examples of people that he thought should not be here. He showed a photograph of a man in the United States whose legs and part of his torso were amputated. Van den Berg also knew such a severely deformed patient. "In response to a letter I addressed to a colleague about an almost maximally deformed patient," he wrote, "the patient had sadly passed away." Without restraint, he continued: "…Sadly passed away! The least it could have said was that no one was able to shed many tears at his death. Or simply: the patient is no longer alive."[79]

---

78   J.H. van den Berg, *Medische macht en medische ethiek*, Nijkerk, Callenbach, 1969, p. 27-28 [Medical power and medical ethics]

79   Van den Berg, op. cit., p. 30

Traffic accidents killed and injured more people in the 1960's than they do today. In Van den Berg's opinion, such people are better off dying. He presented the example of a seventeen-year-old victim: "Perhaps the girl, once awake, will exhibit very severe mental deficiency. She may have permanently lost all interest in life. She may have lost all memories, permanently, from her childhood years up to the accident. It is also possible that, years later, she will exhibit symptoms of a more or less psychopathic life pattern. She may become a thief. She may end up in sexual aberrations. The physician holds nothing back. Is it even permissible to hope the girl will wake up? The parents, supported by the physician, decide it is not. The girl is given a lethal injection. Not that the latter is already taking place: the new code of ethics is still too young. But it will. It must."

Van den Berg outlined a novel way to deal with victims of traffic accidents. "We can expect that, in addition to the AAA road service, there will be something like an organ patrol, in let's say red-colored vehicles, always prepared at the site of an accident, not to help, but to cut the living organs out of the bodies that are at death's door on the spot." These days, the people who cite Van den Berg as their great inspiration do not quote this paragraph very often.

The essence of Van den Berg's new code of ethics can be summarized in one concise paragraph. Today's physician is better able to keep people alive than ever before. However, not everything that is possible is also desirable. Now equipped with new medical techniques, the physician has become all-powerful. Limits must be set to what he does. The physician must act only when there is some meaning to it. If treatment is pointless, the physician will discontinue the treatment or kill the patient. Van den Berg is vague about whom the physician consults to make this decision. Whether the person to be killed, if legally competent, has any say in the matter, is not addressed.

Van den Berg's influential booklet bears this striking feature: all of the disabled and ill individuals described are only examples, objects in an argument. Whether they are mentally competent or not, able to speak or not, Van den Berg never gives them a voice. They are merely objects in a display of what medical power can lead to. Look, these people are still alive, but should we be pleased about it? Wouldn't it have been better if the physician had never treated them? Wouldn't it be better if the physician would let them or cause them to die now?

The point Van den Berg tried to make in 1969 was that a distinction should be made between meaningful and meaningless life. How to distinguish between the two? Van den Berg asked the question. "Where is the boundary? I don't believe there is such a boundary. I also do not believe that it will be possible to determine on paper, that is in general, what is meaningless or meaningful in the context of a human life. I think it would be a waste of time to give this much attention. Moreover, it is not fair to the sick and the dying to quarrel about the theory of it. Action is what is needed."[80]

Reading it forty years later, a paradox stands out immediately. Van den Berg proposes to limit the power of physicians by giving physicians the right to kill patients without too much "quarreling." As if giving doctors the right to end lives without being asked does not increase the power of a physician.

Still, his contemporaries did not see it like this. At that time the protest generation regarded Van den Berg as a visionary who wanted to restrain medical technology in order to increase their own responsibility, to stand up against the omnipotence of the medical profession. This man, who wanted physicians to decide what was meaningful and what was meaningless life, was embraced by the protesters.

Years later, ethicist Heleen Dupuis still commends Van den Berg as the man who increased patient participation and curbed the power of the physician. "Not until the 1960s does the thought emerge in the Netherlands that patients are not merely (suffering) objects …but that the patient, even if he is ill, has an opinion and an idea about his own situation and can be considered able to participate in decisions regarding medical

---

80 Van den Berg, op. cit., p. 47

treatments. ....J.H. van den Berg is the first person to openly talk about this issue in the Dutch medical ethics literature," Dupuis wrote in a 1992 textbook on health ethics.[81]

Van den Berg's book set the tone during the first years of the debate about end-of-life decisions. He was quickly followed by more influential thinkers who advocated euthanasia, a concept that was interpreted very broadly in those days. Whether the termination of life would be done at the request of the individual whose life was at stake was not the issue. The most important thing was that the termination of life was believed to be in the patient's interest. It was seldom made clear who determined the nature of this interest. It was very clear that the person who would decide was not always the same person who would die.

The concept of self-determination was irrelevant in those days. Euthanasia's appeal was not based on voluntariness, on participation, or on self-determination, but rather on mercy (or compassion). A person who was so deformed, so ill, so disabled, would be better off dead. If necessary, a physician must be allowed to help him die.

In the early 1970s P.J. Roscam Abbing argued: "If it is true ...that the individual may request voluntary euthanasia for himself, then it is clear that he may also do this for another, out of love for this other person..."[82]

The Dutch Alleingang

The Netherlands was not alone in those years of rapid social change. Death became a subject of discussion in more countries. More openness and honesty with regard to death was also advocated elsewhere. In Great Britain, for example, the rising hospice movement organized places for people to die as peacefully as possible. All over the Western

---

81   Heleen M. Dupuis, A.H.M. Kerkhoff, P.J. Thung, *Voordelen van de twijfel. Een inleiding tot de gezondheidsethiek*, derde, herziene druk, Houten/Zaventem, Bohn Stafleu van Loghum, 1992, p. 24 [Benefits of the doubt. An introduction to health ethics]

82   P.J. Roscam Abbing, *Toegenomen verantwoordelijkheid. Veranderende ethiek rond euthanasie, eugenetiek en moderne biologie*, Nijkerk, Callenbach, 1972, p. 49. [Increased responsibility. Changing ethics regarding euthanasia, eugenics and modern biology]

world, the generation that emerged in the 1960 and '70s generally held a left-wing orientation, an idealist worldview, and a desire to change society accordingly. Only in the Netherlands, however, did this generation embrace euthanasia as part of its program for a better world.

Dutch American James Kennedy explained this *alleingang*, this going-it-alone, as the Dutch faith in putting everything on the table. In the Dutch view, discussing and breaking concealed taboos enabled people to reach solutions together. Talking about it makes it possible to monitor and control what would otherwise happen in secret. "Breaking the taboo on sex and death was good, and therefore abolishing the taboo on euthanasia, which promised less hypocrisy and more openness, would also be a good thing."

Further advancing the Dutch *alleingang* during that period, only in the Netherlands did the distinction between 'passive' and 'active' euthanasia entirely dissolve. This would have far-reaching consequences, as the Dutch example shows. In all other nations, both concepts were used. They were often defined loosely, lumped together, and even interchanged, but the distinction held. The term 'passive euthanasia' would be used when life-saving treatment was discontinued. In the archetypal example, a person is hooked up to machines in the hospital; after turning off the machines, death occurs. That would be 'passive euthanasia' according to this definition. Injecting a lethal dose of medication would be 'active euthanasia'.

In the Netherlands these definitions are now considered outdated; 'active euthanasia' is now referred to simply as 'euthanasia.' 'Passive euthanasia' is called 'abstaining from treatment'. In other countries the terms 'passive' and 'active euthanasia' are still used. Regardless of what they are called, it is important to make a distinction between the two.

In the Netherlands the euthanasia movement achieved a breakthrough when the public accepted the moral equivalence of passive and active euthanasia. That 'passive euthanasia', i.e. abstaining from treatment, was permissible, was quickly beyond dispute in the Netherlands of the 1970s and 1980s. At that time many regarded technology with suspicion, and people were starting to put quality above quantity in many areas of life. It made sense that people rejected technical tours-de-force that increased the duration, but not the wellbeing, of an individual's life.

But foregoing treatment, even if this leads to death, is accepted in many countries. A certain skepticism against endlessly continuing treatment is also present outside the Netherlands. However, only in the Netherlands did it result in accepting euthanasia; it was only here that 'passive euthanasia' also led to 'active euthanasia'.

Partly responsible for this development was Harry Kuitert, a member of one of the largest Protestant churches in the Netherlands. A well-known theologian, Kuitert has played a major role in the euthanasia debates for thirty years, and has broken other social taboos as well. He provided the deciding push by declaring both forms of life-shortening action morally equal in a book published in 1981.[83] Put crudely: if you shut down the machines, thereby causing a person to die, you achieve the same effect as if you actively kill the person. It makes no difference. And since shutting down the machines is permissible, you are also allowed to actively kill.

This line of reasoning has been used so often and sounds so reasonable that it probably still convinces many people. Yet it remains merely an 'end-justifies-the-means' argument. This 'effect ethic' that examines only the morality of the goals achieved is the opposite of the 'action ethic' that looks at the morality of the action itself. An immoral act can never become morally acceptable because of the higher goal that is achieved by it. Human rights start from an 'action ethic'.

Kuitert, however, quickly gained quite a following with his view that, if abstaining from medical treatment is allowed, then so is active killing. Theo Boer, an ethicist at the Protestant Theological University, described the unexpected consequences of Kuitert's position in a 2007

---

83   H.M. Kuitert, *Een gewenste dood. Euthanasie en zelfbeschikking als moreel en godsdienstig probleem*, Baarn, Ten Have, 1981, p. 29 [A desired death. Euthanasia and self-determination as a moral and religious problem]

article.[84] "It is not difficult to imagine the consequences of this redefinition. As most people at some point will have supported the decision to forego further treatment of a severely suffering patient in a terminal stage... the suggestion is raised that all of us sometimes gloss over 'euthanasia'."

Kuitert's argument denied the difference between 'passive' and 'active' euthanasia and made active euthanasia acceptable. The Health Council, an important government advisory body in the Netherlands, was quick to follow Kuitert's new definition. The two largest Protestant churches also adopted Kuitert's views, and denied any difference between termination of life and abstaining from life-prolonging treatment.[85] Now merged into the Protestant Church in the Netherlands, these two churches took a leading position in the Dutch euthanasia debate.

This is remarkable: in the Netherlands euthanasia was won not from, but largely by Christians. In the early years in particular the Protestants led the call to accept euthanasia. Kuitert, Ekelmans and Muntendam, and later Dupuis, were Protestant euthanasia pioneers. Opposition to euthanasia was found mainly in the Roman Catholic church and among orthodox Protestants. In amazingly plain language, the Jewish author C.I. Dessaur also cautioned against accepting euthanasia.[86]

The Pendulum From Self-Determination To Compassion

With the Netherlands liberal turn about 1980, a new concept was introduced that proved to be of essential significance: self-determination. Man must be allowed to make his own decisions, whether it concerned the economy, faith, sexual orientation or moment of death. This liberal shift also influenced the euthanasia debate. The theme of compassion for people who would be 'better off dead' vanished into the background, replaced by the right of individuals to decide they would rather die.

---

84   Theo D. Boer, Recurring Themes in the Debate about Euthanasia and Assisted Suicide, in: *Journal of Religious Ethics*, 35, 3 (2007)

85   Euthanasie en pastoraat, 1988 [Euthanasia and pastoral care]

86   Dessaur, C.I. and C.J.C. Rutenfrans, Mag de dokter doden? Argumenten en documenten tegen het euthanasiasme, Amsterdam, Querido, 1986

As the debate took place in the media and the public at large, the issue was defined as the autonomous human being who wanted to be able to decide for himself whether he continued to live or not.

This emphasis on self-determination was entirely compatible with the type of euthanasia in which the person makes a request to die: 'termination of life on request'. Self-determination was less compatible with termination-without-request of the lives of people who haven't asked for anything but are suffering severely. Whereas the 1970s discussion was about euthanasia 'in the interest' of a person who did not ask for it, in the 1980s it was all about euthanasia at the express request of the patient. In the 1980s, euthanasia was more narrowly defined than in the 1970s. In 1985, a State Commission on Euthanasia formulated a new definition of 'euthanasia': "intentional life-terminating acts by someone other than the person involved at the latter's request."[87] Since then there has been clarity in the Netherlands: an intentional death was euthanasia only if the dead person had asked for it.

The coma patients, the severely suffering newborns, the people with dementia, were dropped from the picture. From now on the debate would be limited to people who were capable of expressing their will, and who were able to ask for euthanasia.

In this way the euthanasia movement linked up with the 1980s revival of the Western tradition of autonomy and self-determination. Many people in the 1970s still looked to the authorities to realize the dreams of an ideal new world, but in the '80s the government was called upon to step back and let the people shape their own lives. The euthanasia movement, at this point advocating voluntary euthanasia only, dovetailed with this wave of liberalism. Whereas discussion of euthanasia originally began as a form of social criticism of the excessive use of medical technology, it had become right to decide your own end of life. Euthanasia was made into the *magnum opus* of Dutch liberalism in the 1980s. The left-wing liberal democrats (D66) successfully became the champions of euthanasia. It was D66 Member of Parliament

---

87   Report of the Netherlands State Commission on Euthanasia, 1985

Wessel-Tuinstra who in 1984 introduced a first bill to legalize euthanasia (an effort which failed).

The *Dutch Association for Voluntary Euthanasia* (NVVE) also restricted its efforts to people who were competent to ask for their own death. The NVVE also advocated drawing up an advance directive, in case a person becomes incompetent later. Yet termination of life for those who were already incompetent, who were unable to draw up an advance directive or express their will in another way, was not proposed by the NVVE or others.

In the mid-1980s, the Supreme Court accepted euthanasia in the Netherlands. The public regarded it as a form of self-determination. The Court, however, explicitly rejected self-determination as a legal reason for euthanasia. The highest judge stressed that if the suffering of a patient became so severe that a physician ended up in a situation of necessity, that physician was allowed to opt for euthanasia as the lesser of two evils.

When you see films, read commentaries in the newspapers or hear the comments of average people about euthanasia, you can see the depth of the current confusion. Most people think euthanasia and assisted suicide are legal rights in the Netherlands. However, euthanasia is not a 'right' that citizens have. Rather, it is a 'right' that physicians have to meet a request for euthanasia by a citizen, if the physician is of the opinion that their patient suffers. These two things are completely different.

This gap between what the Dutch think about euthanasia and the legal reality has two consequences. First, there have been clashes between patients and physicians because the patients think they have the right to demand euthanasia and physicians are not always willing to comply. Second, the public, with its single-minded focus on self-determination, is oblivious to the debate between physicians and lawyers about termination of life without request for legally incompetent patients.

It should come as no surprise that physicians and citizens clash regularly. In 2005 the NVVE, now renamed *The Dutch Association for the*

Voluntary End of Life, published a book of experiences of surviving relatives. The relatives were often disappointed because the physician did not help their loved one die, or did not do so soon enough.[88] This frequently leads to recriminations. The NVVE therefore demands a broader application of euthanasia, in order to do justice to the citizen's autonomy and to bring actual practice closer to what citizens have been thinking of as their right for a long time.

Physicians, on the other hand, sometimes feel pressured by patients who demand euthanasia. Margriet Oostveen reported in the newspaper *NRC Handelsblad* that after the Euthanasia Act was passed in 2001, family physicians observed a change in the attitude of their patients. "It is as if the law has pushed us doctors across a boundary," said Berdina Wanrooij. "Patients now claim the right to euthanasia, the patient no longer requests to die, he demands it. This was never our intention."

While the public was amazed that a physician could ignore the personal request of a competent patient, they barely noticed the debate that physicians, lawyers, and finally also politicians, initiated in the 1990s about termination of life without request. In the 1980s the public at large as well as the expert elite focused on euthanasia, but since about 1990 the public debate and the expert debate have diverged. Even today the public debate continues to focus mainly on questions of euthanasia and suicide by people who are able to make their own decisions. The elite, in the meantime, is back where they started in the 1970s: are we allowed to decide that someone else, someone who is not heard in the matter, is better off dead? Cases such as this are much more difficult to assess: newborns, for example, or people in a coma, or persons with mental or multiple disabilities. The liberal arguments, based on self-determination by legally competent individuals, are not very helpful here.

A Clear Boundary

---

88   Hans van Dam, *Euthanasie. De praktijk anders bekeken*, Veghel, Libra & Libris, 2005 [Euthanasia. A different perspective on euthanasia practice]

"Non-voluntary euthanasia is murder or manslaughter." Plain language from the mouth of Professor Leenen, an influential proponent of euthanasia in 1977. "The strict enforcement of this standard is in the interest of the individual, but also in the general interest, that consists, among other things, in the fact that the sick and disabled in our society do not have to feel unsafe because decisions can be made about their lives without their input. Crossing this boundary is sometimes permitted in the literature, albeit under strict conditions. However, from the perspective of the law and the right to self-determination, one should not accept any deviation from the principle that euthanasia can never be carried out without the consent of the individual in question."[89] Leenen was not alone; since the 1980s the supporters of euthanasia have frequently stated loudly and clearly that euthanasia would be allowed only for people who asked for it. No one should fear that decisions are made about other people's lives, no one need fear termination of life without request.

Leenen, who died in 2002, devoted his life to describing the rights of patients, and always emphasized self-determination. "Because man as a human being has the right to self-determination, it is irrelevant to which degree he can exercise this right to self-determination …minors and disabled individuals also have the right to self-determination, even if they are limited in actually exercising it. Their right to self-determination must also be respected and every effort must be made to realize it to the degree possible …if deciding one's fate were not the right of the individual, others would be authorized to do so." [90] And that would be unacceptable, because "man's right to self-determination is the basis of euthanasia."[91]

A few years later, however, Leenen wrote the opposite: "It cannot

---

89 Leenen, H.J.J., *Euthanasie in het gezondheidsrecht*, in Muntendam (ed.), Euthanasie, Leiden, Stafleu, 1977, p. 85. [Euthanasia in health law]

90 H.J.J. Leenen, Handboek gezondheidsrecht. Deel 1. Rechten van mensen in de gezondheidszorg, Houten/Diegem, Bohn Stafleu Van Logchum, 2000, fourth edition, p.32-33 [Dutch Health Law Handbook. Part 1. Rights of persons in healthcare]

91 Leenen, ibid., p. 306

be ruled out that unasked-for termination of life through the active intervention of the physician is sometimes justified. This may occur when the patient is unresponsive, is suffering severely without the prospect of improvement and when no alternative pain relief is available. An example is a metastasized cancer process in a non-responsive patient in the terminal stage of the disease, with untreatable severe pain and shortness of breath that threatens to lead to suffocation. The physician can then be caught in such a conflict of duties that he may proceed to termination of life in this exceptional case."[92] He can then claim a situation of necessity. Leenen, who always put self-determination first, still arrived at termination of life without request sometimes being justified to avoid suffering.

The Protestant theologian Harry Kuitert is another person who used plain language. If the killing was not a "killing on request, then we are dealing with murder or manslaughter and that is one of the most immoral (and also punishable) acts a person can commit," he clearly stated.[93] Tampering with this would mean toying with the faith in physicians, he added sternly. "Termination of a person's life is only permitted 'on request'; 'not on request' is not permitted. Fidelity to this principle is the only way to prevent grandmother becoming afraid of her grandson who is a doctor and a member of the *Dutch Association for Voluntary Euthanasia*."

Kuitert continued: "Does this mean that (physicians and hospital teams) must keep alive all people who are not able to express themselves (yet)? I would say: yes, why not? Who would enter a hospital with confidence or watch his relatives go in there if such a question was answered in any other way than with a whole-hearted and unqualified yes?"[94]

---

92   Leenen, ibid., p. 314

93   H.M. Kuitert, Een gewenste dood. Euthanasie en zelfbeschikking als moreel en godsdienstig probleem, Baarn, Ten Have, 1981, p. 29 [A desired death. Euthanasia and self-determination as a moral and religious problem]

94   Ibid., p. 64-65

Plain language from Kuitert: "The only thing we need to add is that there may come a moment when medical treatment becomes pointless because none of the remaining options will contribute to the wellbeing of the patient involved." Kuitert advocated discontinuing or abstaining from treatment if it was medically pointless. This was already normal medical practice, and did not sound very spectacular. He asked "Everything beyond discontinuing or not starting a medically pointless treatment is therefore not permissible?" His answer: "That is correct, I feel we cannot emphasize it enough. Which is not necessarily contrary to physicians sometimes going further." This last sentence sounds odd; is termination of life without request unacceptable or not?

"In one of the last chapters I will talk about stopping resuscitation attempts or discontinuing – or not starting – the treatment of newborns." In those chapters Kuitert wrote about resuscitation: "A condition for starting CPR is the willingness to admit failure and act accordingly. Within the boundaries of this assessment model, switching off the ventilator or even ending a life cannot be worse (more reprehensible) than never starting resuscitation."[95] For the 'severely defective' newborns about whom the decision is already made not to treat them it is also sometimes permissible to kill them: "…when letting die peacefully implies that a severely defective neonate must wait months for certain death, it would appear possible to me that a physician ends such a life gently by administering certain medications, without him incurring any moral damage. He does not harm any interests, because there no longer are any. We could say the reverse: he does the parents and the hospital a service by carrying out a jointly made decision."[96] Here we see that termination of a life without the request of the individual concerned is approved.

In this example, where he condoned termination of life without request, Kuitert justified it by referring to the interests of the hospital and the parents. Not those of the child, because the child no longer had

---

95   Ibid., p. 117
96   Ibid., p. 123

interests, Kuitert argued. The discrepancy with what he argued previously could not be greater.

Apparently it is difficult, once you start, to limit termination of life to the person who asks for it, even if people express in no uncertain terms that they want these limits. Kuitert joined the choir of people who were ambivalent about the question whether termination of life without request is allowed or not. First he resolutely said no, and only pages later said yes.

In 1993 Kuitert wanted to revise his twelve-year-old book on euthanasia, but it quickly developed into a new book that addressed termination of life without request much more extensively.[97] It was still a blessing, Kuitert argued, that in the Netherlands we had defined 'euthanasia' as termination of life on request. However, this did not mean that there can never be termination of life without request. "We merely 'postponed' discussing it" Kuitert now stated.

"The much-needed discussion about termination of life had been limited (by this definition, GvL) to a discussion about termination of life on request. On the one hand this – as I indicated – has rendered euthanasia not only discussible but also morally, legally and politically feasible in the eyes of a large part of our society. From this perspective we can only be grateful for society's adoption of the definition. …Other types of termination of life were mentioned of course, but were systematically excluded from the discussion in order not to confuse the issue."[98] So, in order to "not confuse" the discussion, he had presented euthanasia as termination of life on request. Now that euthanasia was an established concept, Kuitert felt that the time was right to resume the discussion about termination of life without request that had been defined away earlier.

Although this Protestant ethicist claimed in his preface that his thinking had remained largely the same in those twelve years, he now

---

97   H.M. Kuitert, Mag er een eind komen aan het bittere einde? Levensbeëindiging in de context van stervensbegeleiding, Baarn, Ten Have, 1993 [Can the bitter end be ended? Termination of life in the context of terminal care]

98   Ibid., p. 14

proved to be a pronounced supporter of termination of life without request. A patient who is about to die can request euthanasia. Such a request "simplifies the decision-making for the physician," Kuitert wrote, "He knows what the patient wants, the ball is in the patient's court, so to speak." But then Kuitert continued: "But if the patient has no more initiatives because he is too far gone, the physician does not automatically lose his medical responsibility; on the contrary, he takes over from the patient and determines, sailing on the compass of his profession, whether the hour of the bitter end has arrived and when he is convinced it has, he will help the patient depart, even without the patient asking him to. That is why he is a physician. Shocking? Again: is the alternative, in terms of mercilessness, not more shocking?" Note the change: the early Kuitert, who referred to termination of life without request as murder, and the later Kuitert, who felt that termination of life without request is the duty of the physician. The only similarity between the two is the certainty of the theologian's statements. Incidentally, he did not mention whether grandmother would be wise to now fear her grandson who is a member of the euthanasia association NVVE.

Another person who joined the euthanasia debate in those early years was the Baroness H. van Till-d'Aulnis de Bourouill. At that time she was the secretary of the *Foundation for Voluntary Euthanasia [the stichting vrijwillige euthanasie]*, not to be confused with the *Dutch Association for Voluntary Euthanasia* NVVE. She called euthanasia a human right. In an interview with newspaper *Trouw* in 1984 she clearly cautioned against non-voluntary forms of termination of life: "The point is that huge amounts of enormous problems are solved silently, quickly and cheaply by letting die or killing. Killing the weak and the sick, that is. The temptation to let things get out of hand is therefore immense." Her conclusion: termination of life must remain limited to those who ask for it. This supporter of euthanasia did not hesitate to caution against Nazi-like practices, should the boundary to non-voluntary euthanasia be crossed.[99]

---

99 Secretaris van de Stichting Vrijwillige Euthanasie: "Nieuwe wetgeving is onnodig," *newspaper Trouw*, February 20 1984 [New legislation is unnecessary]

At the same time, however, she did not rule out the possibility of non-voluntary euthanasia in some cases. In the case of the mentally handicapped termination of life must be possible, not because of their mental defectiveness, but because of "circumstances extremely difficult to bear," such as pain, shortness of breath, itching, giving off a stench etc. "It is not, it would appear to me, unreasonable to think that he [the mentally disabled person, GvL] suffers as much due to such circumstances as we do."[100]

It is not a crime that the Baroness Van Till-d'Aulnis de Bourouill, theologian Kuitert and health care lawyer Leenen changed their minds. There is no shame in first arguing against and then in favor of the possibility of termination of life without request. People have the right to change their minds. It would have been better, however, if they had explained why they changed their mind and why, on reflection, their earlier warnings regarding non-voluntary termination of life were apparently no longer valid. But they don't. All three of these euthanasia champions first argued against termination of life without request, only to subsequently argue in favor of termination of life without request, without explaining why they changed their minds.

Apparently, accepting the practice of termination of life on request results in also accepting the practice of termination of life without request. Even people who initially vehemently oppose it eventually accept termination of life without request.

In the 1980s the *Dutch Association of General Practitioners* (LHV) also seemed to be speaking plain language about euthanasia. Their opening paragraph was very clear: "In our opinion the element of voluntariness must indeed be present, or the risk of manipulation will be too great. It is inconceivable that another person than the individual concerned makes such a far-reaching decision."

---

100 Quoted in W.C.M. Klijn, Wetswijziging euthanasie wordt een onhoudbare discriminatie, *newspaper Trouw*, June 25 1986 [Euthanasia amendment becomes an untenable discrimination]

But then the GP association added "With regard to newborns and young minors there is the problem that they have never been able to express their will. Leenen feels that terminating the life of newborns is therefore unacceptable. This point of view is too extreme in our opinion. In certain situations the parents should be allowed to make the decision for the child." Then the LHV went further: "Regarding comatose patients and particular categories of demented elderly, we feel that life-terminating action is only permitted when there is sufficient indication that the person concerned – if he were capable of expressing his will – would have wanted his life to be terminated."[101]

This is a contradictory line of reasoning. After stating that euthanasia must only be allowed on request, that the danger of manipulation would otherwise be "too great," the LHV immediately listed categories of legally incompetent individuals who do qualify for termination of life without request. They never addressed how to prevent the manipulation that they were so concerned about just one paragraph earlier.

In the 1970s the *Dutch Association for Voluntary Euthanasia* (NVVE) also used seemingly plain language. On closer inspection, it turned out to be just a little less plain. In 1978 a commission led by NVVE chairman Professor P. Muntendam concluded that "the distinction between voluntary and non-voluntary (i.e. unrequested) euthanasia does not coincide with the distinction between permissible and non-permissible euthanasia, and also that voluntary euthanasia clearly borders on non-voluntary euthanasia. The commission does not, however, consider it part of its assignment to address this issue in more depth in this report."[102] Translated freely: sometimes non-voluntary euthanasia can be permissible – it follows naturally from voluntary euthanasia – but let's not go into that now.

---

101 *Rapport van de Staatscommissie Euthanasie*, Den Haag, Staatsuitgeverij, 1985, dl 3, p. 76 [Report of the Netherlands State Commission on Euthanasia]

102 Rapport van de adviescommissie wetgeving betreffende toelaatbare euthanasie, uitgebracht aan de Nederlandse Vereniging voor Vrijwillige Euthanasie, 1978, p. 34-35 [Report from the advisory commission on legislation regarding permissible euthanasia, presented to the Dutch Association for Voluntary Euthanasia NVVE]

The Warning From Two Dissenters

The inevitable inclusion of non-voluntary euthanasia is exactly what two dissenters on the *State Commission on Euthanasia* cautioned against in 1985. In that year, the commission produced an important recommendation. Euthanasia should only be permitted under very strict conditions, concluded the majority of the commission, and only when people request it.

But this will create problems, argued dissenting commissioners Klijn and Nieboer in their minority report. In no time you will also see termination of life being applied when there is no request, they predicted: "This is quite understandable. Empathy with those persons who are unable to express their will forces itself on us. It is impossible to convincingly defend the strict application of the criterion of freedom – especially in the long run – to those people who experience this as discrimination against those who are unable to express their will." In other words: why should legally incompetent individuals suffer when the competent are allowed to request euthanasia? If one group can request a gentle death, the other group should also get it – even without request.[103] If you don't want termination of life without request, you should not embark on euthanasia, cautioned the two dissenting voices on the *Netherlands State Commission on Euthanasia*. For beware: one will lead to the other.

The Netherlands State Commission on Euthanasia

Klijn and Nieboer failed to convince the rest of the commission; the majority of the 1985 state commission felt it would prove possible to allow euthanasia without ending up with unrequested termination of life. That is definitely not allowed, the commission stated resolutely, only to proceed to make – in the same report - one exception: patients in an irreversible coma may be killed without request.

It is evident that a person in a coma, or in a persistent vegetative state, is unable to ask for euthanasia. Yet the commission wanted to

---

103 Report of the Netherlands State Commission on Euthanasia, 1985, p.253

make euthanasia possible for coma patients, even though they could make no request. The majority of the commission proved the minority warning correct. This illustrates how difficult it is to limit euthanasia to people who ask for it.

Even though the majority in the State Commission advised that euthanasia should be possible, the Netherlands' physicians' association KNMG objected that this does not go far enough. They referred in 1985 to the requirement that the State Commission placed on the request as "extreme" and "rigid." It would never be possible to end the life of people who were not in full possession of their faculties, the KNMG responded to the State Commission. "We do not consider such an extreme and rigid position to always be in the best interest of the categories of patients in question [the incompetent, GvL]. If one would wish to create some room for these poignant cases where it is plausible to presume that the patients in question would have chosen euthanasia had they been able to express their will, then it would appear inevitable to us, that others must be granted some right to decide." The KNMG physicians saw themselves and the family as the deciding authority for these cases.[104]

Even as physicians and euthanasia supporters were already beginning to discuss forms of termination of life without request, the public discussion in the Netherlands in those years was limited definitively to the much simpler theme of euthanasia on request. The *State Commission on Euthanasia* defined euthanasia in this limited sense. That was its biggest achievement; after 1985 there was no longer any confusion of concepts in the Netherlands. The term 'euthanasia' referred only to active termination of life at one's own request. Euthanasia, now limited to the voluntary cases by definition, made its definitive appearance as the symbol of self-determination of the articulate individual.

Another Judicial Breakthrough

In the same period the judiciary was responsible for another definitive breakthrough. On November 24 1984 the Supreme Court of the

---

104 Report by State Commission on Euthanasia, 1985, part 3, p. 74

Netherlands opens the door to euthanasia in the Netherlands in the *Schoonheim* case.

A 95-year old woman who experienced her suffering as unbearable was killed at her own request by her physician, Dr. Schoonheim. Initially the physician was acquitted by the lowest court, the District Court. On appeal, the Court of Appeal decided differently, and the physician was convicted, albeit without being given a punishment.

Then the Supreme Court sprang into action. This highest court decided that the Court of Appeal had wrongly convicted the physician, and set aside the judgment of the Court of Appeal. The highest court said that the Court of Appeal should have investigated "whether, according to accepted responsible medical practice, and tested against the standards prevalent in medical ethics, this was a situation of necessity, of *force majeure*."[105] The physician can find himself in a 'situation of necessity' due to the conflicting duties of being bound to alleviate pain on the one hand, and preserving life on the other, the Supreme Court found. Because of this 'situation of necessity', the physician was found not guilty, even though the law does not allow euthanasia.

With this decision, the Supreme Court made history. Not the legislators, but the judges made euthanasia possible in the Netherlands. It took another seventeen years for the legislators to follow with the Euthanasia Act.

How did the highest court in the Netherlands arrive at this breakthrough? The Supreme Court referred to "accepted responsible medical understanding, tested against the standards prevalent in medical ethics." During the same months that the Supreme Court examined this case, this medical understanding changed, because the board of the physicians' organization KNMG issued rules regarding euthanasia. This U-turn by the physicians influenced the judiciary in the *Schoonheim*

---

105 Supreme Court November 27 1984, *NJ* 1987, 608

case, as Attorney General Remmelink argued.[106] The KNMG changed its mind, and because the judges looked at what was medically accepted, the judges then also change their minds.

It is remarkable, however, that the *Royal Dutch Medical Association* KNMG pointed out that physicians were very much divided. The association did not really want to comment on whether or not euthanasia should be allowed. "This is not about questioning the permissibility of euthanasia," the KNMG wrote in its 1984 position on euthanasia.[107] "In a plural society like ours there will always be different opinions on the issue, also in the medical profession. ...The commission and the executive board started from the fact that euthanasia is actually carried out." The KNMG then presented a few 'due care' requirements for physicians who planned to carry out euthanasia. Paraphrasing what the KNMG said: physicians are divided about whether euthanasia is acceptable, but because some of the physicians carry out euthanasia regardless, we will at least draw up some rules, which does not mean that the KNMG approves of euthanasia.

This view quickly proved too subtle to survive in the real world. As soon as you formulate rules for something, you automatically propose that you agree with whatever happens according to those rules. The highest court in the Netherlands promptly took this medical profession's divided position as a reason to assume that "according to accepted responsible medical understanding" a physician is sometimes allowed to carry out euthanasia.

All-in-all, euthanasia had its breakthrough in the Netherlands in 1984. The highest court based its decision in this important case partly on the about-face of physicians' association KNMG. The physicians' association cautioned: "...first and foremost must be that the request for euthanasia is based on the free will of the individual involved..."

---

106 Matthijs de Blois, *Een juridisch perspectief*, in: P.J. Lieverse (et al.), *Dood gewoon? Perspectieven op 35 jaar euthanasie in Nederland*, 2005, p. 62 [A legal perspective, in P.J. Lieverse et al., Dead normal? Perspectives on 35 years of euthanasia in the Netherlands]

107 KNMG, Standpunt inzake euthanasie, *Medisch Contact* 39, 1984, p. 990-997 [Position regarding euthanasia]

This sounds resolute, perhaps more resolute than intended. In the introduction of their "position on euthanasia," the physicians' association formulated it slightly differently: "The position is relevant only for those cases in which the patient in question is capable of expressing his will. In view of the fact that the euthanasia issue is both comprehensive and complex, the executive board has imposed this restriction on itself for now." For now, indeed.

An Honest Answer

Several years after the Supreme Court all but legalized euthanasia, physicians started the follow-up discussion: if termination of life on request is allowed, can it then also be allowed without a request? For example, what if a patient was unable to ask for it?

In December 1990 the future Minister of Public Health Els Borst-Ei-lers, member of political party *Democrats 66* (D66), and at that time chair of the *Dutch Health Council*, spoke at a small conference in Maas-tricht. A certain person asked why a request by the person whose life is going to be ended was necessary in the case of euthanasia. After all, he reminded her, the Dutch euthanasia practice is justified by saying that its goal is to alleviate pain. But, the person continued, people who are unable to express their will, people who are unable to request anything, can also suffer. Shouldn't it be possible to end their suffering as well, the person asked, even without request?

Borst answered: "It was a tactic. By starting with this category we could achieve a gradual acceptance of euthanasia." By "this category," Borst meant people who were competent and able to ask for euthanasia. The emphasis on self-determination in the euthanasia debate, Borst admitted, had been a tactic.

The secretary-general of physicians' association KNMG at the time, Th.M.G. van Berkestijn, added that decriminalizing termination of life on request was significant because it prepared the way for cases involving people who were unable to personally ask for euthanasia. "The answer to the question whether the implication is that we would proceed with the non-voluntary cases after euthanasia in the narrow definition had been decriminalized is yes, under strictly limited conditions."[108]

The attending American professor Alexander Morgan Capron observed in his report: "It was an instance, or so it seemed to me, when the candor of our hosts was a little chilling."

A New Commission: *Acceptability of Life-Terminating Action*

But Borst and Van Berkestijn were not exaggerating. At the time of this 1990 conference, a *Commission for the Acceptability of Life Terminating Action* (CAL) of the *Royal Dutch Medical Association* (KNMG) had been at work for a year. This Commission investigated exactly what Borst and Van Berkestijn were publicly referring to. Now that termination of life on request had been allowed by the courts, could we carry out termination of life without request in some cases from now on? The final report was published in 1997.[109]

The medical debate on termination of life without request started by staking out a position. In the preface to the Commission's report, KNMG president professor J.M. van Minderhoud congratulated the physicians on the Dutch open-mindedness that made these discussions possible. "The Commission has demonstrated an acute awareness that it was bringing up for discussion subjects that can be extremely sensitive for some people. On the other hand, a discussion like this is exceedingly stimulating for the sound practice of our profession and we should consider ourselves fortunate that we enable one another to exchange views about these problems."

---

108 This episode is described in Maurice A.M. de Wachter, *Euthanasia in the Netherlands*, Hastings Center Report (1992) 22, 2, p. 23-30. De Wachter organized the meeting of seven Dutch and seven international experts. Also present was Alexander Morgan Capron, who reports on it in *Euthanasia in the Netherlands. American observations*, Hastings Center Report (1992) 22, 2, p. 30-33. John Keown also attended, but for the quotes of Borst and Van Berkestijn he refers to Alexander Morgan Capron, see John Keown, *Euthanasia, Ethics and Public Policy. An Argument Against Legalisation*, Cambridge University Press, 2002, p.149.

109 R.J.M. Dillmann (et al.), *Medisch handelen rond het levenseinde bij wilsonbekwame patiënten*, Commissie Aanvaardbaarheid Levensbeëindigend handelen KNMG, Houten/Diegem, Bohn Stafleu Van Logchum, 1997 [Medical practice around the end of life of incompetent patients]

It is a recurring phenomenon in the discussion of the admissibility of termination of life by Dutch physicians that the participants congratulate each other on their open-mindedness, which the Dutch like to call typically Dutch. But if you think that there are no forbidden ideas in this open Dutch debate, you are mistaken.

Everything Is Discussible – *Except A Different View*

The fact is that the views of the *Catholic Association of Care Institutions* KVZ, for example, were not welcome. The KVZ sounded this warning: "The debate on termination of life without request, to which the medical profession again makes an important contribution, and even takes an important first step via the KNMG commission, feeds into the societal notion that a person's life need not be preserved in case of a certain degree of suffering or a certain perspective and in some cases can be terminated – without request."[110]

This kind of fundamental criticism of both the existence of, and the questions asked by, the *Commission for the Acceptability of Life Terminating Action* (CAL) was brushed aside by the Commission in its preface: "It is not possible to respond to all criticism... In some instances the criticism seemed to suggest that the Commission would have done better not to discuss certain issues at all, almost as if the discussion papers were causing the problems they discussed. ...the Commission is still convinced that the problems it was requested to investigate are very real [societal] problems."

It is astonishing that criticism was rejected so cavalierly. Of course it is true that the Commission was investigating "very real societal problems." The Commission observed that these also occurred in other countries, where they have not led to the conclusion that physicians are sometimes allowed to end a person's life without request. In those countries, no *Commission for the Acceptability of Life Terminating Action* has been set up. One can recognize "very real societal problems" and still be of the opinion that physicians should not kill people without

---

[110] Ibid, p. 7

being asked. The warning of the *Catholic Association of Care Institutions* KVZ corresponded with what is still a common view outside the Netherlands. The warning did not mean that this Catholic association denied the "very real societal problems." However, because this Catholic association had no intention of accepting termination of life without request, and questioned the entire setup of the Commission, the CAL simply decided not to respond to this criticism. Here the CAL demonstrated the limits of how we "enable one another to exchange views about these problems," which is so "stimulating for the sound practice of our profession." Anyone with a different opinion is excluded in the introduction. The entire 'debate' held by the CAL created the impression that the question whether life-terminating action on legally incompetent persons would be admissible had already been answered with "yes."

'Making discussible' apparently means 'making acceptable.' The open debate in reality is only open to those with the correct views. Perhaps that, too, is typically Dutch.

In this way the debate was limited to people who want to move more or less in the same direction. After eight years the *Commission for the Acceptability of Life Terminating Action* came to crystal-clear conclusions. In specific situations it is acceptable to end the lives of people who are not competent, whether they are coma patients, newborns, people with dementia or psychiatric patients. Much less clear than the conclusion were the arguments the Commission used.

Persons In A Vegetative State

Take, for example, the considerations of the CAL regarding patients in a persistant vegetative state, people who have been in a coma and have never regained consciousness. The language used was very difficult to read, but they were saying something important, so it is worthwhile to quote the report here. "If one accepts the analysis that the existence of a patient in a persistent vegetative state is a resultant of an existing life, of a severe condition, and of the medical treatment of this condition and the support of the life, then it is no longer self-evident to appeal to the presence of life in this patient as a reason for continued treatment. For one has contributed to this life being in this specific situation. This means one is at least partly responsible for the consequences of being in this situation. The fact that the patient is alive is still relevant and of great importance, but it is not a sufficient argument to continue treatment."[111] Especially when the Commission uses impenetrable language, it turns out to be taking the biggest steps. As it does here. The essence of the argument is that "it is no longer self-evident that one can appeal to the presence of life in this patient" if the patient is alive only because of earlier medical treatment. This life is therefore less worthy of protection than other lives, especially of people who stayed alive on their own. This life, and the authority to decide whether it should continue, is in the hands of the physician who saved it earlier. He is responsible for this situation because he caused it. The Commission's argument is more alarming when it is clearly stated.

In those days, this line of reasoning was not unique to the Netherlands. The discussion was actually turned backward. It was not termination of life without request that should be questioned, but the preceding decisions to prolong life.[112] This is remarkable. One would expect that termination of life without request is the act that needs legitimizing. This is not acceptable anywhere in the world. It was explicitly declared out of the question in the Netherlands several years earlier, in the 1980s discussion about legalizing euthanasia. Nevertheless, the CAL clearly stated that the physician who ends a person's life without request is not the one who must justify his actions, but rather the physician who decides to prolong a life.

Full circle: the discussion ends up back where it started in 1969, back to the warning sounded by J.H. van den Berg concerning unbridled medical technology. Not every medical technique has to be used, not in every case should life be saved and prolonged. This is reasonable. Medical technology is sometimes not started; treatment is sometimes

---

111 Ibid, p. 99

112 John Griffiths et al., *Euthanasia and Law in the Netherlands*, Amsterdam, Amsterdam University Press, 1998, p. 118 ff

discontinued. This is true both within the Netherlands, and elsewhere. However, Van den Berg's unique contribution to the Netherlands is that if a life is first saved, and subsequently proves to fall short in terms of quality, that life may, if necessary, be actively terminated.

The CAL, however, denied there was anything to explain: "... (it is) unmistakable that this report discusses different categories of patients for whom active life-terminating action must be considered anything but commonplace. This is also the CAL's conclusion: while explicitly recognizing that opinions on this matter vary within the Commission and the medical profession, active life-terminating action is only conceivable in exceptional situations."

Hidden behind the reassuring remark that life-terminating action must be seen as "anything but commonplace" and that the medical profession is divided on the subject, this document clearly states that it is allowed. "The problems were not, however, created by the Commission and denying them is obviously pointless. In this context it is of the utmost importance to address the [technological] developments in medicine. More important, however, is that the Commission holds that the primary question is whether continuing medical treatment is legitimate, especially when this treatment can be regarded as merely prolonging life and it has little to no positive effects for the patient. With this position we do not want to focus on the question when active life-termination action can be acceptable, we wish to pursue an ethically desired limitation of medical action."[113] The *Commission for the Acceptability of Life Terminating Action* appears to be reasoning that advancing medical technology creates the problems, that medical treatment sometimes leads merely to prolonging life without having positive effects for patients.

It is one thing to say that not every medical technique should be applied every time. It is quite another to say that if those technological developments don't provide good results, physicians are sometimes allowed to kill the patient. Yet the Commission decided that the latter follows from the former.

---

113 Op.cit., p. 26

It is clear that self-determination barely factored into the considerations of the CAL. This might seem logical, because the CAL focused on incompetent people, who might be unable to express their will. Anyone who has an "incompetent" person among his relatives or friends, also knows that a person who cannot speak well or is mentally challenged is sometimes quite capable of expressing his likes and dislikes. However, the physicians on the *Commission for the Acceptability of Life Terminating Action* wrote that even the patient who was still capable of making decisions about his own life could be ignored.

Read what physicians had to say about people who awaken from a vegetative state. "The only reason one could have to continue treatment is the ... minimal chance that the situation will change, and the patient will regain consciousness. It is assumed that this is also what the patient in question wants. However, it is far from evident that the person actually wants this, because regaining consciousness in these cases is unfortunately always accompanied by severe disorders and restricted possibilities to give shape to one's own life." The CAL touched on a real issue here: waking up from a coma is sometimes portrayed too optimistically in the media, as if the person simply picks up where he left off. This is not reality; often there is permanent damage when someone wakes up. So how might we assess the quality of life of the person who has regained consciousness? "The persons involved should be the first to speak on the subject. Nevertheless one may consider whether those individuals who have come out of a vegetative state – had they been able to make a decision – would have chosen differently. Once consciousness has been regained, it is hard to give it up, even though one would have rejected the situation as undesirable beforehand. The frequently occurring personality changes complicate the assessment of whether the situation would have been different if there had been a possibility to choose."

First the CAL says that the people involved, the persons who have come out of a vegetative state and now live with impairments, must decide. This is the language of self-determination. Yet then the remainder of the paragraph says exactly the opposite – it is *not* up to the people involved to decide. The first sentence merely pays lip service to the self-determination of former coma patients. In the rest of the argument this self-determination turns into its opposite.

Now awake, the former coma patient does value his life – but he is not who he was before. If his former self could have decided, he surely would not have wanted this. Therefore, the Commission stated, we must not hold out too much hope that coma patients or people in a vegetative state will wake up. If they do wake up, they will have brain damage. If they feel that their life is valuable despite the injury, physicians wonder if they should attach any importance to the opinion of a disabled person. Worth repeating, because it is nothing short of cynical, is the sentence: "Once consciousness has been regained, it is hard to give it up…"[114] The Commission, however, has not yet arrived where it wanted to go.

It concluded that a moment may come when further treatment of a patient is not justified. But, if further treatment is pointless and death is expected, is active termination of life also legitimate? The arguments for and against active termination are set forth impressively. Yet when it comes to the conclusion, a brief sentence that did not weigh the previous conflicting arguments was enough for the Commission: "In light of the second approach – which carries an important grain of truth – the Commission is of the opinion that active termination of life after all medical treatment is abstained from, which will inevitably cause the patient to die, is not necessary but should also not be categorically rejected." The Commission listed the arguments for and against termination of life and drew the conclusion that the arguments in favor of termination of life are stronger. It did not explain why. Surely we may regard that as odd.

After this important conclusion the Commission appeared to put on the brakes. Physicians who are not willing to actively kill coma patients, don't have to, the Commission said reassuringly. However, this does not mean their patient will then live: "The Commission observes that there are physicians who cannot accept administering pharmaceuticals in deadly dosages on moral grounds. If, from the perspective of adequate help in dying, it is decided that this is still necessary (and opinions

---

114 Ibid., p.100 ff.

diverge) then it is recommended to organize an adequate referral or transfer of the treatment."[115]

Here we have a legally undefined concept, 'adequate help in dying'. Apparently it means that if a physician refuses additional treatment to an incompetent patient, the physician could consider killing the patient by 'administering pharmaceuticals in deadly dosages.' Clearly, this is termination of life. The Commission of the physicians' association also observed that the physicians, "opinions diverge" on whether this is acceptable. Without explaining why, the Commission concluded that the physicians who reject termination of life as not acceptable must yield to the physicians who feel that it is.

The situation could have been reversed. Given the division, the Commission could have concluded that the physicians who feel that termination of life is acceptable must renounce it because they are unable to convince all their colleagues. Without any explanation, without consideration, the Commission opted for the other path: termination of life must be made possible, and the dissenters must resign themselves to it.

Dementia

People with dementia eventually become incompetent, and can then no longer request euthanasia. Are there any specific situations that would allow them to be killed? The physicians' Commission asked the question.

Many people with dementia live in nursing homes. Euthanasia and termination of life are rare, as geriatric physicians in the Netherlands are very reserved when it comes to life-terminating action. The *Association of Geriatric Physicians* NVVA rejected termination of the life of people with dementia, purely on the grounds of their loss of competence. Only if the demented patient contracts another severe illness would geriatric physicians imagine ending the patient's life – in extreme cases.

The *Commission for the Acceptability of Life Terminating Action* weighed in: the geriatric physicians did not go far enough. The Commission

---

115 Ibid., p. 104

noted "...that the NVVA rejects the possibility of active euthanasia based on 'only' the presence of a (severe) dementia, even when the patient has a euthanasia directive." It was the Commission's opinion "that the categorical rejection of active termination of life based on a severe dementia does not resolve this complex ethical issue." This is a peculiar sentence. The referral to "this complex ethical issue" in itself is not an argument for termination of life. One could argue equally that living with dementia is a real "complex ethical issue," one which is not resolved by termination of life. You can contend either position, but in both cases it comes down to the arguments. And we do not get to read those.

When terms like "complex ethical issue" are used, they sound impressive and suggest that physicians have pondered the issue and proceeded carefully. This creates the illusion of care. On closer inspection the physicians lack arguments. Without arguments their conclusion that 'termination of life must sometimes be allowed' is simply a claim suspended in a vacuum. To the superficial reader, however, the conclusion appears to have been reached carefully.

One thing the geriatric physicians' association and the Commission agreed on was that abstaining from further treatment can sometimes be acceptable in the case of dementia. The Commission urged that the 'quality of life' added by the medical treatment should be examined. The term 'quality of life' is controversial, because it implies a value judgment about another person's life. If the term was not used, on the other hand, treatment could be continued and life prolonged, with no benefit to the patient. The Commission proposed the compromise of not looking at the dementia patient's quality of life, which obviously is not the physician's domain, but to look at the quality that the proposed medical treatment adds to the patient's life. "The life of the demented elderly person is the measure used to determine the added value of medical treatment. The measure itself is not subject to assessment, however."[116]

The Committee's conclusion: abstaining from treatment is allowed. But will that make the next step – to actively terminate the life of a

---

116 Ibid., p. 123

person with dementia – acceptable in the future? The Commission answered this question in small steps, shifting its position slightly each time, until nearly every category of people with dementia, with or without a euthanasia directive, was made eligible for termination of life.

The first small step considered a hypothetical patient who had drawn up an advance directive stating he wanted to be euthanized if he became demented. Under certain conditions, they concluded, such a patient could indeed be killed, as would be confirmed later in the 2002 Dutch Euthanasia Act. Self-determination was the justification, and once again it proved to be a strong argument for allowing euthanasia.

In the second step, the Commission looked at people with dementia who did not draw up a euthanasia directive in the past, but who had expressed their will in discussions or notes that could now be reconstructed. The Commission felt that if other symptoms besides the dementia indicated severe suffering, ending the lives of severely demented patients was conceivable. Here the Commission made an attempt to respect the will of the person involved, albeit in a roundabout way.

However, in the third step, the Commission went on to state that even the life of a person with dementia who has never asked for euthanasia or termination of life in an advance directive, or never said or recorded anything from which such a desire could be reconstructed, could be terminated 'in a situation of necessity'. "The Commission is of the opinion that in these situations the presence of a severe dementia is an insufficient precondition for life-terminating action. The situation must at least be one of obvious necessity in which the patient's situation is in conflict with human dignity, and the suffering of the patient cannot be averted in an acceptable manner."[117]

But what does 'in conflict with human dignity' mean? Why is 'conflict with human dignity' so bad that it would justify killing such people without their request? Two pages later, the point was formulated slightly differently: "If there is neither an advance directive, nor a convincingly

---

117 Ibid., p. 139-140

reconstructed personal will, a ground for life-terminating action could perhaps be found in the intention to end a situation that is evidently appalling and in conflict with human dignity."

Now another criterion appears out of nowhere without explanation: 'evidently appalling', in addition to the earlier mentioned 'in conflict with human dignity'. Obviously the physicians were not formulating real criteria here, but marshalling important sounding words that could be used interchangeably at will.

Psychiatric Patients

Most cases of suicide involve people with psychiatric disorders, according to the Commission.[118] Should a physician be allowed to assist a person with a psychiatric disorder to end his life? People who suffer from such a disorder may be incompetent. There is a chance that their will-to-die is a result of their disease.

In the paragraph entitled *The legitimacy of the physician* the Commission formulated its reasons why the physician should be allowed to help a psychiatric patient kill himself. Again, the wording is confused, but the Commission ended with a clear conclusion. It is worthwhile to read the entire argument, quoted below.

"However, in the treatment of a psychiatric patient it may become clear after a considerable period of time that it is not successful: the condition can perhaps be influenced, but it recurs more frequently and more severely, or the condition (and related symptoms) cannot be treated satisfactorily. In the context of such a long-term treatment relationship, the nature of the perspective of healing, and keeping death at bay, may change. This prior involvement in the treatment in particular, or an important part of it, can provide the moral justification for the psychiatrist to have a role in assisted suicide. The Commission notes that apart from moral justification, there are medical-professional aspects that should be considered. We will return to this point in detail later. In its discussion paper the Commission pointed out an additional fact, namely that the

---

118 Ibid., p. 146 ff

physician is the only person who can give the patient access to drugs, i.e. the physician is the keeper of the key to the medicine cabinet."

"The Commission does not want to assign any decisive moral significance to this fact, even though it determines part of the actual role physicians have. The primary legitimacy of the involvement of the physician can be formulated like this. Medical knowledge and experience indicate that suicidal patients must be treated. However much we may expect or hope for improvement, treatment is not always successful. Nevertheless, because of this expectation and hope, patients have been treated many years, with a temporary or a limited result. If, after expert treatment, it must be acknowledged that from a medical point of view no healing (of the death wishes) can be offered, and the patient now expressly requests assistance in ending his life, then the legitimacy to do so is located in the prior medical history. In the opinion of the Commission it is deemed acceptable that in those exceptional instances the psychiatrist could provide assistance in the suicide. However, the Commission expressly does not consider this the duty of the psychiatrist, although it understands that some psychiatrists might experience it as such."[119]

This is not a very logical argument. The next-to-last sentence contains the conclusion at issue. Psychiatrists are allowed to assist their suicidal patients to kill themselves if they have been treating the patient for a good while and are having no success.

Certainly, the psychiatric patient may be mentally incompetent. In that case, assisted suicide is not acceptable, the Commission acknowledged. Then this paragraph. "A psychiatric patient who suffers severely and has a persistent, enduring desire to die, and whose suffering cannot be averted in an acceptable manner, may perhaps not meet the most stringent requirements regarding mental competence. The Commission does not deem this fact decisive: if there is no treatment perspective, the patient suffers severely and unavoidably, and the patient expressly and repeatedly wishes to die, then the application of the most stringent requirement of mental competence is cruel. It should be considered that,

119 Ibid., p. 150

by making this requirement as a physician, one aggravates suffering instead of warding it off."

So, of the stringent requirements regarding assisted suicide, the requirement of mental competence was abandoned in one paragraph because it is supposedly "cruel" to hold onto the requirement. Again, it is clear how easily compassion or pity replaces self-determination when it comes to justifying termination of life.

Sometimes psychiatric patients are placed in psychiatric hospitals involuntarily to prevent them from hurting themselves. This is regulated in the *Psychiatric Hospitals Compulsory Admission Act* [*Wet BOPZ*]. It may appear contradictory that psychiatrists lock people up to prevent them killing themselves, and subsequently help those people kill themselves. The CAL was of the opinion that this was acceptable. The Commission did add that the obvious course of events would be to first release the patient from the admission and then assist him with his suicide.[120]

Compassion? or Paternalistic Pity?

In a word, unrequested termination of life is permissible. According to the Dutch Medical Commission that studied the issue in the 1990s, this is not as sensational as it might initially seem. Life-terminating action on people who did not ask for it is one of many possible medical decisions that are relevant towards the end of life. CAL indicates that often the prior decision to forego or discontinue treatment is more important than the subsequent termination of life.

The *Commission for the Acceptability of Life Terminating Action* followed the argument presented by theologian Kuitert in 1981 – there is no substantial difference between the physician who decides not to continue treating a person and to let him die, and the physician who decides not to continue treatment and to actively terminate his life. Is the effect, CAL asked, not the same?

---

120 Ibid., p. 169

The Commission's justification for unrequested termination of life was 'compassion', although the physicians' Commission sometimes preferred to refer to it as 'mercy'. Whenever physicians believe that terminating life in specific situations is acceptable, they intend to end the suffering of the incompetent patient. In those cases in which the patients are able to ask for it, self-determination is considered an important justification for euthanasia. Yet if a patient is unable to ask for termination of life, physicians could proceed with it by referring to the need to reduce suffering. From a legal perspective the physician's compassion toward his patient is a key in the Dutch justification of euthanasia. The physician must determine that the patient's suffering is hopeless and unbearable.

In the end, the Dutch euthanasia practice, with or without request, is based on compassion or mercy, not self-determination. Euthanasia supporters in other countries who appeal to self-determination should therefore be asked: how they avoid what happened in the Netherlands from happening in their countries?

Chapter 7

Abstaining From Treatment

Accepted Medical Practice And Death

Termination of life receives a lot of attention, but death can be brought closer by less visible medical decisions. A physician may abstain from medical treatment, for example, because he feels it would be medically futile. This is considered normal medical practice.

In the public Dutch euthanasia debate, the value of life was openly discussed. The same controversies about the value of life can be seen in the discussions over abstaining from medical treatment. When something as radical as termination of life is acceptable in a country, it will be much less problematic to decide to abstain from treatment.

Of course 'discontinuing treatment' does not mean that the physician does nothing for his patient. The physician stops the life-prolonging treatment, and replaces it with a treatment that aims to let the patient die as peacefully as possible, says Armand Girbes, professor and ICU-physician at the Amsterdam VU medical center hospital. "Actually, physicians should never stop treating a patient. However, the treatment goal may be changed. The original therapeutic goal of total cure or prolonging life may be changed into optimal palliative treatment, when it becomes clear that the patient has reached the end of his life."[121]

Advocates of the possibility of life termination like to point out that it can be difficult to distinguish among the possible decisions made just

---

[121] Armand R.J. Girbes, End of life decisions in the ICU. A Dutch perspective, *Care of the critically ill*, 2006, 22: p. 1-2

before the end of life. The decision that all treatment options for that patient are exhausted, and to refrain from further treatment is at least as important as the possible subsequent decision to terminate that person's life. In this way, it has been argued that termination of life is less shocking than it would appear to be at first glance. "Don't get all worked up about termination of life," the argument goes. "Instead, get worked up about the previous decision to stop treatment, because that is the essential decision."

But this argument raises questions. Who decides that life-saving treatment of a patient is pointless? And on what grounds? If a patient is capable of deciding that he does not want the treatment, the situation is clear: the patient gets his way, and the treatment is either discontinued or never started. However, a decision not to treat can also be made by the physician - against the wishes of the patient or his family - if the physician judges the treatment to be medically futile.

A physician can decide that a treatment is medically futile if the treatment has no chance of being successful. This is the clearest form of medical futility: it won't work, so there is no point. The treatment is also referred to as prospectless.

Although the treatment itself might be successful, a treatment can also be called medically futile if the costs are not in proportion to the benefits. 'Costs' refer not only to the monetary costs of the treatment, but also to how burdensome the treatment is to the patient.

A third possibility is that a treatment could be successful, but the physician still deems it 'medically futile', because 'a certain minimum level' can no longer be achieved.[122] In their Health Law textbook, the Netherlands' future medical lawyers will read: "Due to the nature of the illness or defect the patient is severely affected or damaged and there is little or nothing the doctors can do to improve this, or there is a tragic cumulation of ailments and defects that could, through a disproportionate effort, perhaps be treated separately, but together in their totality

---

[122] H.J.J. Leenen, J.K.M. Gevers, J. Legemaate, 2007, op. cit., p. 321-322

are not or almost not treatable." As the verbosity suggests, this type of medical futility is the most difficult to determine. There are no rules. The physician has to judge each individual case separately.

This gives physicians a certain kind of power. They have the right, based on their professional knowledge, to decide what is medically futile. This right is unreservedly theirs. On several occasions judges have made it clear that the physician, not the family, decides what is medically futile. In one case, when their child suffered a severe brain injury, the parents wanted life-prolonging treatment. The physician refused to put the child on a ventilator; the courts backed the physician.[123] Many other pressing issues face physicians. Is it medically pointless to give nutrition and fluids to a person in a persistent vegetative state? If so, does the physician alone make the decision?[124] This does not automatically mean that physicians will always decide to withhold food and fluids from these patients.

We must ask an important question: how does a physician reach his decision? Remember – only if a physician submits a report that he has actively ended a person's life, will his actions be reviewed. On the other hand, it is considered normal medical practice for a physician to abstain from treatment, even if his decision results in the patient dying of his disease. No report is required, the doctor's actions are not scrutinized, and no special requirements of due care apply.

Could a physician's decision that treatment is 'medically futile' perhaps be a cover for something else? This rhetorical question was asked by British legal scholar and critic John Keown.[125] Sometimes, Keown stated, 'futility of treatment' is confused with 'futility of life'. In particular, this confusion occurs when the decision not to treat is based on the 'future quality' of the patient's life, as anticipated by the physician.

---

[123] Decision by the president of the Court of Utrecht in interlocutory proceedings, January 11 1991, *Tijdschrift voor Gezondheidsrecht* 1991/28

[124] H.J.J. Leenen, J.K.M. Gevers, J. Legemaate, 2007, op. cit., p. 328

[125] Keown, John, *Euthanasia, Ethics and Public Policy. An Argument Against Legalisation*, Cambridge University Press, 2002, p. 243

Imagine the cases of two children with comparable multiple disabilities, who develop pneumonia. After consulting with both sets of parents, the physician decides not to provide antibiotics to either child. The first child continually swallowed the wrong way due to its disabilities, and as a result contracted pneumonia over and over again. That would be a medical reason. The second child had no swallowing problem, and the pneumonia occurred only once. Still, it was not given antibiotics. Apparently there is a different, non-medical reason at work in this case. Clearly, it makes a difference whether the physician bases his decision on medical facts or not.

ICU Physicians of the Rotterdam Erasmus Medical Center do not look at the prospective quality of life their patient will enjoy if they save his life. This concept is simply too subjective, according to intensive care clinical ethicist Erwin Kompanje. Physicians do not have a crystal ball to predict the quality of a person's life. According to Kompanje, physicians should decide whether a life-saving treatment is medically indicated based on medical facts. A guideline adopted in 2009 by the *Netherlands Society of Intensive Care* (NVIC) regarding foregoing or discontinuing treatment leaves no room for decisions based on the patient's quality of life. Only two acceptable reasons exist for discontinuing, or not initiating, a treatment, declared the NVIC: either that treatment is futile, or the costs and burden of the treatment outweigh its benefits.

But the public debate on medical decisions sometimes reflects how the decision about the futility of a treatment becomes intertwined with the futility of a life. The distinction between the two is not always easy to make.

Should We Treat The Baby With Down Syndrome?

Should a baby with Down syndrome get the same medical treatment as a baby that does not have Down syndrome? In 1988 and 1989 this subject was hotly disputed in the Dutch media. This debate concerned the birth of a child with Down syndrome, who also had an intestinal obstruction. An operation could fix the intestinal obstruction. Down syndrome, however, cannot be cured. The parents decided not to have the operation for their child, and the child died very soon afterwards. The child received no treatment because the parents felt it was better that the child died.

The story became known nationwide as the *Baby Ross* case after the treating physician, J.C. Molenaar, published an article about it.[126] Under the title *Medicine, Servant Of Compassion [Geneeskunde, dienares der barmhartigheid]* this pediatric surgeon recounted why he decided not to operate on the baby. The parents of the child were both of the considered opinion that it would be better if it died, because "their child would never grow up to be an independent individual; institutionalization was a real possibility…" The family's physician disagreed with this decision, filed a protest and informed the Public Prosecutor. The prosecutor temporarily entrusted the child to the care of child protective services. Eventually, respecting the parents' decision, the *Dutch Child Welfare Council (Raad voor de Kinderbescherming*, RVDK) decided not to order the surgeon to perform the operation. These are the facts of the case.

Pediatric surgeon Molenaar did not choose neutral words to recount these facts. Although his article opened with the usual professional language, the surgeon shifted to more emotional words as he described the deathbed of the child he did not treat: "In the days that followed both parents surrounded the child with the highest degree of care and attention until it died in his mother's arms four days later. After the baby died the parents personally tended to and laid out the child." He could have given a factual description: "The parents stayed with the child until it passed away," but he did not do that. He chose to use positive, emotive language like "the highest degree of care and attention," "in his mother's arms," and "personally tended to and laid out."

As it happens, the combination of Down syndrome and intestinal obstruction is not uncommon, and Molenaar had a very similar case in the

---

126 J.C. Molenaar, K. Gill, H.M. Dupuis, Geneeskunde, dienares der barmhartigheid, *Nederlands Tijdschrift voor Geneeskunde* 1988; 132, p.1913-1917 [Medicine, servant of mercy]

same week. In this case, the parents decided that their baby should have the operation. Again Molenaar respected the decision of the parents, and treated this child. In his description, however, Molenaar chose very different words: "This child is alive and will grow up as a mongoloid patient." The difference with the lovingly described baby one paragraph earlier is remarkable. When parents of a Down baby let their child die, their physician chooses warm words to describe the harmonious end of the child. Conversely, when parents decide on treatment for their child with Down syndrome and therefore to let him live, he chooses to say that this child "…will grow up as a mongoloid patient." This formulation is neither factual nor neutral. The physician would have been factual and neutral had he written: "This child will grow up with Down syndrome."

Superfluously, the physician added this prognosis: "Not one single patient with this syndrome is capable of surviving independently in society. Many of them will have to live in institutions. Some will be able to live at home, but due to early onset dementia considerable problems could develop there."

According to Molenaar, the essence of the matter is that medicine must reduce suffering, not increase it. This is in line with "the principle of mercy and compassion as the basis for human action." In the words of ethicist Heleen Dupuis, who collaborated on Molenaar's article and supported his actions: "Had their baby been born twenty years ago, everyone would have breathed a sigh of relief and said: fortunately it is not viable. Today it is not either, unless we intervene. We decide not to, as this will only cause more suffering, and that is not what medicine is there for."

The sentence "as this will only cause more suffering" is very telling. The thought that apart from suffering, the life of this child with Down syndrome could also have brought happiness, for the child and for the people around it, never enters Dupuis' mind. According to her, living with Down syndrome only brings "more suffering."

When they were criticized in the Dutch physicians' journal *Nederlands Tijdschrift voor Geneeskunde*, Molenaar and Dupuis revisited the question whether parents could decide if a child with Down syndrome should be treated or not. "The value of a human life is determined by what others feel it is worth," Dupuis and Molenaar argued. The parents are the ones who decide whether the child lives. "Considering the ill newborn rather than the parents as the person asking for assistance, is therefore not realistic. Those who claim that it is only make a rhetorical contribution to the discussion."

The decision to treat should only be made when the treatment is in proportion to the expected result, argued Molenaar and Dupuis. The language they used was ostensibly academic: "This applies especially when, with a maximum application of medical possibilities (neonatal surgery and perioperative neonatal intensive care) the outcome with certainty is a mentally subnormal life (i.e. a patient with Down syndrome). If an operation is the only way to save a mentally defective life, the point and acceptability of such an operation may therefore be called into question."

Stated in everyday language: If after the surgery and intensive care, the child still has Down syndrome, we may question whether the operation should have been carried out.[127]

Philosopher Paul Cobben, who has a son with Down syndrome, responded in the newspaper *Volkskrant*. After the birth of his son, he secretly hoped that his son had a defect that would cause him to die quickly. He, his wife, and the people around them agreed that they had been struck by disaster. "Trained in the tradition of enlightenment I regarded freedom and free will as the supreme good. And my son was going to be an inferior, imperfect human being." Six years later, in 1989, Cobben wrote: "The question whether he is a human being now seems absurd to me. He is proud when he has learned something new, he can be super excited when he gets to play football, he can comfort people

---

[127] Nederlands Tijdschrift voor Geneeskunde, 1989; 133, p. 86-91

when they are sad, he is embarrassed when he wets himself, and so on. But it's true, he will never be an ethics professor."[128]

Professor of ethics Dupuis responded to this statement, recounting how many furious reactions she received. These are people who don't understand, she declared. Not everything should be done simply because it is possible. "Sometimes it is better to let a child die," particularly if the child and his family will suffer severely if the child lives. Does Dupuis know how to decide between certain present death and possible future suffering? "I don't know, nobody knows." For this reason, Dupuis argued, it should be the parents' decision. If they choose to abstain from treatment and consequently to let their child with Down syndrome die, then this is their right.[129]

Paul Cobben pointed out that if one follows Dupuis' argument, parents of a Down child could also simply stop feeding the child to cause its death. "Based on this argument it is permitted to let all mongols die, as long as it is with the consent of their legal representative."

Health jurist and professor H.J.J Leenen, joining the discussion, recognized that physicians must navigate another kind of confusion. It was acceptable, he argued, to weigh the goal against the means. It was acceptable to abstain from treatment if very aggressive treatment will have a relatively limited result. It would not be acceptable to abstain from treating the Down syndrome child because of the supposed insufficient quality of the child's life. "In my opinion nobody – including the parents – has the right to judge whether he thinks a person is good enough to receive a necessary medical treatment. And it is wrong in my opinion to withhold the treatment, that is given to everyone else, from the baby because it has Down syndrome."

Heleen Dupuis constructed yet another argument to support the parents' 'right to refuse treatment' for their child with Down syndrome.

---

128 Paul Cobben, Medische opvatting is voor mongolen levensbedreigend, *de Volkskrant*, March 18 1989 [Medical view is life-threatening for mongols]

129 Heleen Dupuis, Soms is het beter een kindje te laten sterven, *de Volkskrant*, April 8 1989 [It is sometimes better to let a child die]

Perhaps to reassure us, she introduced this argument by stating the exact opposite of her planned conclusion: "The death of a newborn is no less painful that the death of an adult." Yet then she stated that the lives of babies are less worthy of protection than the lives of others. "When a newborn doesn't make it, this is not the same as when, for example, the mother of a young family dies."

The life of a baby, according to Dupuis, is therefore less worthy of protection than the life of a person who is older. In other cultures, she wrote, the killing of unwanted children shortly after they are born has always been common practice. "Fortunately we are more humane in how we treat our most vulnerable fellow human beings." Yet in her opinion 'humane' sometimes also meant that you should not save a newborn, for example, because it has Down syndrome.

A weak argument, according to Leenen. We have established human rights that determine that all human beings are equal from birth. A baby has just as much right to life as an older human being. This is a legal decision that cannot be ignored; if you are born, you are a human being and all human beings are equal.

In the late 1980s the courts ruled in the *Baby Ross* case about the non-treatment of the child with Down syndrome. The Public Prosecution Service had decided to prosecute the surgeon involved, among others. This did not develop into a criminal case: the idea that such prosecution is not reasonable had been accepted all the way up to the Supreme Court.[130] The key argument was that because the treatment could have caused much suffering, the physician had the right to decide against treating the child. According to an expert witness, professor Vos, the fact that the child had an intestinal obstruction could be an indicator of additional physical defects. Vos described children with Down syndrome who did receive treatment as follows: "This included children

130   The procedure was different because the people being prosecuted objected to the decision of the PPS to prosecute them. As a result the court only marginally reviewed whether prosecution was reasonable. According to the judges it was not, which is why criminal proceedings were never commenced.

whose suffering defies description. I can only describe their lives as deeply tragic... Taking stock I can only say that the situation these children will end up in is an ocean of horror." As a result the Den Bosch court spoke of the great risk that the operation would open the door to a life of very serious suffering for both child and parents.

The Den Bosch court indicated that the interest of the child was not the only consideration in the decision to treat or not – the interest of the parents must also be included. Jurist and critic G.W. Brands-Bottema pointed out that a person's right to protection of his life would now be weighed against the degree of suffering that his life might bring to third parties.[131] If another person suffers due to the fact that you exist, then your life is less worthy of protection.

Still, this argument is not uncommon. At about the same time of the Den Bosch court decision, the *Commission for the Acceptability of Life Terminating Action* (CAL) also considered whether parents have the right to decide on the death and life of their child. When it involves a child who is heading for an 'unlivable life', according to CAL, the parents do have the right to decide whether their child receives medical treatment. On the other hand, the CAL physicians argued, it also depends upon the parents' acceptance of the child, and on the degree of effective care they can provide to a child with an 'unlivable life'. Sometimes it is acceptable for physicians to decide against treating a disabled child if, in the physician's judgment, the parents will not care for it properly. One way or another, whether the child is permitted to live or not, the decision depends upon the parents – or on the physicians' assessment of the parents.

Rightly so, the physicians argued: "It is their child after all, they are the most closely involved, relationally and by law and – after the child itself – they also have the greatest interest in the decision that is to be made. After all, if the decision is to let a severely defective child live, the far-reaching consequences of this decision are to be borne not by the treating physician(s), not by the hospital administrations, but by

---

131 Dorscheidt, op. cit., p. 227

the parents (as well as the child and other members of the family)."[132] Responding to the controversy over the term 'unlivable life', the physicians' committee replaced it with 'prognosis regarding state of health' in a later version of the report. However, their position remained substantially the same.

Even the pediatricians in those years argued that parents should have a say in whether a child with Down syndrome should be treated or not. The report *To Act Or Not?*, by the *Dutch Pediatric Association* NVK, mentioned the example of a child with Down syndrome who has an additional problem, such as an intestinal obstruction, that will cause the child to die if it is not treated. The physicians were divided, but the majority decided: "If they are informed parents, who reach their decisions carefully, who are convinced that a surgical correction will not benefit their child and their family, this opinion must be respected. Even if the medical team doubts the correctness of the decision, even if the treating physician would make a different decision for his own child, this is still a situation in which many sensible citizens in our plural society would decide against an operation. If he pushes through a therapy the parents do not want in such an uncertain situation, the physician exceeds his authority." So, if parents are well informed, if they make a careful assessment, they can decide that a necessary treatment is not in the interest of the child and the family, and that it is therefore better to let their child die.[133]

The Value Of Life With Disability

Another area in which the value of a life with disability is questioned is the situation of very premature babies. Difficult decisions must often be made in the care for these children. If the decision is to abstain from medical treatment, a child dies. If the baby is treated, it might survive but the risk of disabilities is considerable. Whereas previous

---

132 *Levensbeëindigend handelen bij wilsonbekwame patiënten. Deel 1: zwaar-defecte pasgeborenen.* Discussienota KNMG-commissie aanvaardbaarheid levensbeëindigend handelen, Medisch Contact 43 (1988), p. 697-704 [Life-terminating action in incompetent patients. Part 1: severely defective newborns]

133 *Doen of laten?*, op. cit., p. 46 [To act or not]

chapters discussed the issue of termination of life in babies, which is not very common but very controversial, here the issue is abstaining from treatment after which the child dies a natural death – less controversial, but much more common.

Eric Vermeulen visited neonatal departments to study decision making surrounding babies that are born extremely prematurely in a Dutch and a Flemish hospital. He observed that, as soon as disabilities were anticipated, physicians acted as if further treatment of a baby had no chance of being successful. Although the proposed treatment might have positive results, physicians would declare that treatment futile if the surviving baby would be disabled. "Even if the child could survive after continued therapy, this option is not really offered."[134]

Vermeulen focused on the way the physicians spoke and the arguments they used, both among colleagues and with the parents. Vermeulen quoted a neonatologist who was treating a child born after a pregnancy of only 25 weeks and three days. If the physician treated the child and it lived, it would probably be affected. The physician said: " … this is a child that we need to find arguments for to refrain from treatment." When the sonogram turned out positive, the neonatologist concluded: "Now you end up in the treatment circuit." Once there, it is very difficult to stop treatment: the child was saved, but the doctor's question lingers: should it have been?

These are real dilemmas in neonatology. One important study followed approximately 1,300 children who were born with a birth weight under 1,500 grams and/or before week 32 of the pregnancy. Since 1983, 28 percent of them died in the first year. At the age of five 13 percent had an impairment and 14 percent had a disability. Twenty percent had behavior disorders. At age nine 19 percent of the children attended special needs schools. Estimates by the Dutch National Health Council suggested that forty percent of the children who would still be alive in the year

---

134   Eric Vermeulen, *Een proeve van leven. Praten en beslissen over extreem te vroeg geboren kinderen*, proefschrift Groningen, 2001, p.265-266 [A test of life. Talking and making decisions about extremely premature babies. Dissertation]

2000 would have problems leading independent lives in society when they became adults.[135]

Different countries handle these risks differently. Dutch physicians exercise more restraint than their colleagues in other countries.[136] Some Dutch parents turn to German hospitals as soon as they suspect their child will be born very prematurely, because they want to ensure the best possible chance that their child will be treated.[137] The guideline in the Netherlands is to treat prematurely born babies from week 24. In practice, however, Dutch physicians are more reserved. They do not always treat children in the 25th week either, as research from 2008 shows.[138] The decision to treat or not is related to the risks of disabilities the physician is willing to take.

Research into all infant deaths on intensive care units in the Netherlands between October 2005 and September 2006 shows that in 58 percent of the cases the babies had no chance of surviving. The remaining 42 percent might have survived, but their physicians, expecting a 'low quality of life', decided against life-saving treatment. The same study of deaths on pediatric ICUs shows there has been only one case of active termination of life. Abstaining from treatment is obviously much more common than active termination of life.

What makes the anticipated 'quality of life' of these babies so sad that physicians decide not to treat them but to let them die? In the study, the most frequently mentioned reason is 'anticipated suffering'. The future suffering rarely means 'pain'; instead, it means 'anticipated

---

135 *Ibid.*, p. 86

136 See also R. de Leeuw, M. Cuttini, M. Nadia, I. Berbik, G. Hansen, A. Kucinskas, S. Lenoir, A. Levin, J. Persson, M. Rebagliato, M. Reid, M. Schroell, U. de Vonderweid and other members of the Euronic Studygroup. Treatment choices for extremely preterm infants: An international perspective. In: *The Journal of Pediatrics* 2000; 137: p. 608-15

137 Zu jung zum Leben? *Die Zeit*, August 28 2008 [Too young to live?]

138 J.A. Gerrits-Kuiper, R. de Heus, H.A.A. Brouwers, G.H.A. Visser, A.L. den Ouden, L.A.A. Kollée, Op de grens van levensvatbaarheid: Nederlands verwijsbeleid bij vroeggeboorte te terughoudend, *Nederlands Tijdschrift voor Geneeskunde* 2008; 152: p. 383-388 [On the edge of viability: restraint in Dutch referral policy in premature babies]

suffering due to functional impairment'.[139] "Our findings confirm that future quality of life is of crucial importance for Dutch physicians. They are willing, exclusively on the basis of anticipated quality of life, to abstain from or discontinue life-extending treatment," wrote the researchers, including the Groningen pediatrician Eduard Verhagen.[140]

Of those premature babies who died untreated because of a poor prognosis, all of the parents agreed to it. Sometimes they did not agree immediately. In those cases the physicians gave them more time and information, until agreement was reached after all.[141]

Is Surviving With a Disability a Failure?

Are disabled people better off dead? Not many people will answer "yes." And yet the same question, in a veiled way, is sometimes answered affirmatively.

In a 1994 article Heleen Dupuis argued that a physician must remedy pain or at least not increase suffering. She furthermore argues that the costs of medical treatments should be weighed against their benefits. This sounds reasonable. It is important, however, to note that she uses a broad definition of 'costs': she includes disabled life in the category 'costs'. For Dupuis, disabled life includes only suffering and not happiness, consists only of costs, with no benefits.

Dupuis, a senator for the free-market libertarian party VVD, illustrated her argument with the example of resuscitation of two people. One person comes out of it perfectly healthy, but the other survives with

---

139 Op. cit., p. 61

140 A.A.Eduard Verhagen, Jozef H.H.M. Dorscheidt, Bernadette Engels, Joep H. Hubben, Pieter J. Sauer, *End-of-life decisions in severely ill newborns in the Dutch NICU*, in: A.A.E. Verhagen, *End-of-life decisions in Dutch neonatal intensive care units*, dissertation Rijksuniversiteit Groningen, 2009, Zutphen, Paris Legal Publishers, 2008, p. 55

141 A.A.Eduard Verhagen, Mirjam de Vos, Jozef H.H.M. Dorscheidt, Bernadette Engels, Joep H. Hubben, Pieter J. Sauer, *Differences of opinion regarding end-of-life decisions in severely ill newborns in the NICU; results of a nationwide study in the Netherlands*, in: A.A.E. Verhagen, *End-of-life decisions in Dutch neonatal intensive care units*, diss. Rijksuniversiteit Groningen, 2009, Zutphen, Paris Legal Publishers, 2008, p. 65-79

disabilities. This is very nice for the first person, according to Dupuis, but we must also include the cost of the one who survives with severe disabilities. "The appropriate starting point is that there must be no risk of death of a person who could have survived in good health. However, there is a big problem here. Because those who survive, not in good health but severely disabled, actually pay the price for the healthy survival of the group that does turn out alright." Here Dupuis describes healthy survival as valuable. On the other hand, those who survive resuscitation with serious disabilities, according to her are victims of the life-saving treatment. "Should the resuscitation that resulted in a continuation of the life of the patient, but a disabled life, be qualified as a success?," Dupuis asks. "Probably, if the criterion is that the death of the patient was prevented; if, however, the criterion is that a person can live on in a relatively good state of health, then obviously not." [142]

Perhaps, one might object, the resuscitated person who is severely disabled by the trauma is happy to be alive. Dupuis did not consider this possibility. Although she contended that a rescue is a failure if the survivor is disabled, she did not offer even one argument in support. Apparently, Dupuis felt this was so obvious that no explanation was necessary. Dupuis did not think to ask disabled persons who owe their lives to resuscitation how they rate their life with their disabilities. If they were unable to speak, she did not bother to observe them to see whether they seem to be happy.

Dupuis clearly follows J.H. van den Berg, the founder of the euthanasia movement in the Netherlands. In the pamphlet mentioned earlier, Van den Berg presented disabled persons as objects that serve only to prove his argument that medical treatment sometimes yields the most peculiar failures.

The first problem with Dupuis' argument is that she reduced the disabled to silent objects. Second, and even more problematic, was her application of an almost economic assessment of costs and benefits, of

---

142 H.M. Dupuis, Wel of niet behandelen? Baat het niet, dan schaadt het wél, Baarn, Ambo, 1994 [Treat or not treat? It does hurt to try]

suffering and happiness, to human beings. If you cost more than you yield, if you cause more suffering than happiness, you are better off dead. In Dupuis' world, human rights would not apply to people whose lives bring distress to themselves and others.

On the intensive care unit (ICU) of the Erasmus University Medical Center in Rotterdam Erwin Kompanje expressed amusement at Heleen Dupuis' proposition that people who survive with severe disabilities after a medical intervention "are paying the price" for people who leave the hospital in good shape. If the objective of medical treatment is to have only healthy people survive, then the ICUs are in trouble. "We might as well shut down," says Kompanje, a clinical ethicist specializing in intensive care. After one year, sixty percent of all the people who are admitted into the ICU are still alive, and of those sixty percent more than one third are profoundly dependent on others.

The Phenomenon of Fear Toward 'Helpless Vegetables'

Resuscitation is often mentioned when the public debate addresses abstaining from treatment. Participants in the debate frequently point out the limited success of attempted resuscitation. "The vegetable phenomenon" as cardiologist Ruud Koster of the Amsterdam AMC hospital calls it: the inclination of the media to always bring up the many people who allegedly survive resuscitation as 'vegetables'. According to Koster, who is closely associated with the *Dutch Resuscitation Council* [*Nederlandse Reanimatie Raad*] this has little to do with reality.

"Two things are often confused when it comes to resuscitation." On the one hand most resuscitation attempts fail: more than eighty percent of the persons who undergo resuscitation, die. On the other hand, the large majority of those who do survive, end up in good shape. The number of people who survive severely disabled, is small. In the public debate the chance that resuscitation is successful but that the person in question faces the rest of his life severely affected by disabilities, is sometimes confused with the risk that resuscitation fails, which is indeed considerable.

"Of the people who survive, eighty percent end up OK," says Koster. "They may have some trouble remembering a telephone number now and then, but other than that their resuscitation has few consequences. Another ten percent sustain considerable injury. Only ten percent survive resuscitation in a really poor condition. It happens, and then you think: 'What a disaster; I wish we hadn't started on this road'."

In the late summer of 2008 a care facility in the city of Amersfoort caused a stir by announcing a 'no, unless' policy: from now on there will be no resuscitation of the elderly residents, unless the residents have indicated in advance that they do want to be resuscitated in the event of an emergency.

But age is a poor criterion, according to Ruud Koster. "Our own figures show that elderly people do not necessarily come through a resuscitation in poorer shape than younger persons. If a ninety-year-old was to have a cardiac arrest in a supermarket, I would not hesitate to defibrillate her. Why not? The question whether life is still worth anything has nothing to do with resuscitation."

The 'no, unless' policy, in which a care home generally does not apply resuscitation, has since been shot down, says Koster. Resuscitation should not take place when people indicate they do not want to be resuscitated. In all other cases resuscitation must be carried out, unless it is medically futile because a person is terminally ill and their organs are already beginning to fail.

If a person survives resuscitation but is left with injuries, sometimes the partner is more bothered by that than the person in question, according to Koster. The partner often is more aware that a person has changed than the resuscitated person himself. Koster is of the opinion that we must act based on the interest of the patient, not his partner. "As a healthy person you should not judge the life of a patient."

Documentary: *I Don't Ever Want To Be Famous*

In 2006 a startling documentary on resuscitation was released in the Netherlands. Mercedes Stalenhoef's film *I Don't Ever Want To Be Famous* [*Ik wil nooit beroemd worden*] raises the question whether it is sometimes better not to resuscitate.

In its compelling beginning, this film documents the life of cellist Tobias – his cardiac arrest, the resuscitation, the coma he fell into, the slow and difficult recovery afterwards. Difficult especially because it will never be a full recovery. Tobias was a gifted cellist in the prime of his life, from a cultured urban environment. Now in his early forties, he is severely disabled, and can no longer play the cello.

Initially the film focuses on Tobias himself, on his profound disabilities, his speaking problems, but also the unremitting pleasure he takes in music, his high spirits. His brother and sister, his mother, his best friend: people around him do everything to keep in contact with him and bring him moments of joy. Tobias himself is sometimes happy, sometimes sad. We see him enjoying the water with a room mate in the swimming pool of the care facility where he lives, we see how fond the room mate and he are of each other.

However, *I Don't Ever Want To Be Famous* gradually changes course, because the viewer is slowly led in a different direction. The perspective shifts to the people around Tobias, the able-bodied people. Living with a son, or a brother, or a friend who no longer is who he used to be is hard, and they show it. "It would have been better if he had died then," Tobias' sister says about the moment her brother became disabled. "Then again, better for whom?" she adds honestly. Because Tobias himself does not seem to be troubled by his disabilities.

Tobias was resuscitated after a cardiac arrest. With hindsight the question is whether this was wise. And the question now is whether he should be resuscitated again if his heart stops again. His family feels he shouldn't be. Tears are cried when Tobias has just been moved to a new home, an anthroposophic care facility where, unlike previous institutions where Tobias was a resident, they do want to resuscitate should Tobias have another cardiac arrest. The mother is inconsolable when she hears this. "Nobody told me that, about their beliefs and that there are so many taboos," she says.

After her film was released, director Mercedes Stalenhoef was interviewed in the newspaper *de Volkskrant*. When she described Tobias, and his move to the new residency that did not reject resuscitation for disabled persons, she chose remarkable words. Before the move, she recounted, the fact that the family wanted no resuscitation for Tobias was no problem. "The move turned it into one, which led to questions being asked about the desirability of termination of life and the meaning of life. Does his life have meaning? Is Tobias happy? Looking at him I see a young man who is relatively happy. But this is not clear-cut, no matter how often Tobias says he is very happy and wants to live to be a hundred years old."[143] "The desirability of termination of life": according to the documentary's director, this is the essential issue. This is the context in which resuscitating or not resuscitating a disabled person is discussed. Stalenhoef was profoundly mistaken: foregoing resuscitation is not considered to be termination of life.

It is one thing to say that life is tough for Tobias and his family. It is something else to say that Tobias would be better off dead. Stalenhoef, however, combines these two things, thus raising the question whether this disabled man would be better off dead. When Stalenhoef subsequently answers this question "yes," she sets the table for the next question: should he, or should he not be resuscitated in the future? The answer to that question is not based upon medical facts, such as the cause of the circulatory failure; Stalenhoef instead considers only the degree of disability of the person who is to be resuscitated.

We may ask many justified questions regarding the use of resuscitation of healthy and unhealthy persons. If help is late in arriving, there may be cause not to initiate the resuscitation procedure, regardless of whether the person with a

---

[143] Jan Pieter Ekker, 'Bach is de beste', *de Volkskrant*, November 24 2005 [Bach is the best]

cardiac arrest is disabled or not. Yet in this film the debate on whether resuscitation still serves a purpose focuses only on the disabled person. Apparently, Stalenhoef believes that some people are not worth saving.

"We all hope that won't happen," his brother says about the possibility that Tobias will have another cardiac arrest. "On the other hand..." Because this is not entirely true, the brother admits: part of him wants Tobias to die. The family refers to the old Tobias. "I am sure this is not what he would have wanted," his sister says. "I am sure he would have said: euthanasia! This is not what I want," says his brother. "Sitting around like this all day every day, not able to read," says Tobias' mother.

Whereupon Tobias himself says: "I don't want to die." Due to his brain damage he has trouble speaking, but this he says very clearly. However, it is not about him here. Everybody is given a chance to speak and the documentary maker probes deeper every time, but when Tobias says "I don't want to die," Stalenhoef asks not a word.

Then again, Tobias is not the central character in this film. The people around Tobias are. The film is not about what Tobias wants, it is about what his environment wants. This environment discusses the desirability of death. Tobias' death, that is.

At the end of the documentary the director has edited several clips together in which Tobias' family and best friend express their doubt about the value of his life, and actually wish him to be dead. This is followed immediately by the film's final scene in which they all sing a song in celebration of Tobias' birthday.

After an impressive, poignant and loving start the film *I Don't Ever Want To Be Famous* changes into a discussion of the desirability of Tobias' death. This makes it very effective. The way the people around him treat Tobias is heartwarming. After the warm, humane beginning you tend to sympathize with Tobias' family and good friend to such a degree that, before you know it, you agree with the way they talk about the value of his life and the redundancy of his resuscitation.

The credits mention that the film is supported by the *Dutch Association for a Voluntary End to Life*, NVVE. The NVVE wants you to ask yourself whether you want to be resuscitated. Tobias exemplifies what could happen if you don't: look, this is what can happen if you are resuscitated. The man with the disability turns into an example, an object in the NVVE argument. It is therefore no surprise that his own opinion – "I don't want to die" – is ignored.

Mercedes Stalenhoef's award-winning film was well received and shown in numerous Dutch art cinemas and on television. Two years after the documentary, in 2008, Tobias passed away in his sleep.

CONTEXT: *"Rik was going to be a little freak in a wheelchair"*

"Had he been my first, I don't know if I would have been vigilant enough. But he was my fifth." Henriëtte van den Noort from the village of IJsselmuiden in the eastern part of the Netherlands talks about the birth of her son Rik in 2003. Rik was born with a severe form of spina bifida. His spine pointed out at an angle of ninety degrees. After the birth, via caesarean section, in a hospital in the city of Zwolle, Rik was transferred to the University Medical Center in Groningen.

Here the parents were told their son could not be treated. The physicians warned them that Rik would experience unbearable suffering. This sounded a little strange to Henriette, because he lay in his bed very peacefully and drank his milk hungrily. The physicians also said that Rik would not be able to sit upright, let alone walk. His mind would be affected. Rik would be "a little freak in a wheelchair," and have "no quality of life." Henriëtte and her husband prepared themselves for the imminent death of their son and they wanted him to die in their arms.

After a short while Rik was given a heavy painkiller. His parents saw it made him drowsy and caused him to stop drinking. "They said he had a life expectancy of no more than three months. "But we won't let it come to that," they added. That's when something shifted for my husband and me." The parents had accepted that their child was going to die, but that the doctors were to decide when, that was too much.

The medical staff in Groningen said that Rik's parents could ask them anything they wanted. "The next day we asked them to stop giving him Tramadol," the medication that made Rik so drowsy he stopped drinking. That request did not go down well with the physician; she said it was a vote of no confidence by the parents. "We were to take Rik to the hospital in Zwolle immediately. We had no travel basket with us, no coat, nothing. The hospital did give us a blanket for Rik." In their own car, with Rik with his open spine on their lap, they drove to the other hospital. "We drove to Zwolle singing psalms and hoping he could die in his own crib," Henriëtte van den Noort, an orthodox protestant, recounts.

For privacy reasons the University Medical Center Groningen was unable to respond to the story of Rik van den Noort's parents, but said "it is extremely regrettable that this is how they experienced events."

Once in Zwolle, it became clear after a few days that Rik could go home. There was still a serious risk that he would die, but he did not need intensive care and could be nursed at home.

To decide what they should do about Rik, his parents asked for a second opinion from an academic hospital in Nijmegen. "This is a Roman-Catholic hospital, and they are a bit more conservative." In Nijmegen they said the best thing was to keep Rik at home and wait to see what would happen; the chance of him dying was estimated at fifty percent.

After several months Rik developed hydrocephalus (water on the brain), which is not uncommon in children with spina bifida. Now you could tell he was in pain, according to his mother. A shunt needed to be placed to drain the fluid from his brain. The neurosurgeon in Nijmegen objected to this course of action, Rik's mother recounts. "He said: "He will need something like fifty operations, do you want to put your child through that? He has no quality of life." He ultimately did undergo the surgery, but only as a palliative measure, to prevent pain."

After that, Rik continued to grow up at home with his parents in Ijsselmuiden. After eighteen months he had gotten so much stronger that he could have surgery on his back. Henriëtte: "The orthopedic surgeon sawed through his back and removed a few vertebrae."

In all, Rik had three operations by the time he was five years old; a fourth operation is imminent. He can sit upright and moves around in a wheelchair. There is nothing wrong with his mind. Henriëtte: "Rik is not a sad little boy, he is always in high spirits and he plays outside with other children in the neighborhood. With my husband he crawls across the floor, to see who is faster. I sometimes wonder what a disability actually is. All of my children have things they are good at and things they are not good at."

CONTEXT: *"The family wanted me not to treat him."*

Prof. Armand Girbes is in charge of the intensive care unit of VU Medical Center in Amsterdam. "A large, athletic man arrived at the intensive care unit after sustaining serious trauma. His lower right leg had been crushed, and he had serious injury to his lungs and abdomen. We felt his chance of survival was good, but we could not save his leg and had to amputate it. The patient himself was unconscious."

Armand Girbes talks about the discussion with the family. "No leg? He is better off dead then," his relatives said. Sport was everything to him, and he had said on occasion that he would rather be dead than disabled." The family did not want him to be operated on, while such an operation would save his life.

"I explained to the family that, in view of the extreme consequences, I needed to hear a refusal to be operated from the patient himself. But this was not possible. I therefore chose to start treatment in the interest of the patient. His family became very aggressive towards me, especially his girlfriend was livid. She said I was arrogant."

"Later, when the patient had left the IC in good physical shape, I asked him how he felt about our decision. He was happy we had saved his life. He was able to compete at the highest level again, now in the disabled sports. No, I did not tell him his girlfriend wanted me to let him die."

"We also had a woman on the ICU with severe pancreatitis. She was very ill, she was on life support, she was swollen and various organ systems were failing. The risk of death for these patients is approximately fifty percent, but if she pulled through she would make a full recovery."

"I enter the ward unsuspectingly when her husband says to me: 'Doctor, we have discussed it with the whole family and we have decided that you must stop the treatment. She is suffering too much.' He brandished a euthanasia directive from the NVVE, signed by his wife, in which she said she did not want to live on as a vegetable. I explained to him that the medical expertise was essential and that her chances of recovery were fifty percent. We treated her and she made a full recovery."

"I think both families acted out of love, it really is out of love that they say these things. And she did look horrible. But the fact that they ask is also a sign of the society we live in, and it is of course quite bizarre. I have both the French and the Dutch nationality; in France relatives don't make such a request. They know it is impossible."

INSET *"I am one hundred percent in favor of resuscitation"*

Drasko Klikovac: "Irena is 29 years old, completely healthy but mentally handicapped. She lives in a home. Irena can be very cheerful, but she can also feel gloomy."

"Initially we had a clear agreement: if her heart stops, she will be resuscitated. But at some point we heard that this had changed: she would now only be resuscitated if her quality of life remained the same. You can't know this in advance and it also gives the impression that they feel her current quality of life really is insufficient. We talked about it and we have now agreed that, if anything happens, she will be taken to the emergency room and the physician there will decide."

"There are 112 residents at the home. Most of the staff don't know how to resuscitate, and the home has no defibrillator. I have offered to buy one together with other parents; including training eight people how to use it this would cost 3,000 Euros. They weren't interested."

"I am one hunded percent in favor of resuscitation, regardless of the quality of life. To me life itself is what matters most, I am religious too. But I do understand parents who do not want resuscitation for their child. They see their child as being unhappy. Or they experience it as a burden. Irena's mother couldn't cope, we were divorced within months after she was born. I can't blame her, I know how heavy it is. But I wanted to take care of Irena myself."

Drasko took care of his daughter for a long time. Now that she is living in a care home, he works the night shift in another residential care facility. "There are residents there whose file says: do not give antibiotics."

Chapter 8

Despair And Arrogance

Why We Make Judgments About Others

The Reason For This Book

I did not write this book out of the blue. I started writing it when circumstances changed me from an average Dutchman who thought of euthanasia as one of the crowning achievements of our liberal country into someone who was shocked by the harsh tone used by the Dutch when they talk about handicapped life.

It started off with a small pea. In 1994, Niek, my partner of six years, was found to have what we called a "small pea" in his head. Sometimes we also referred to it as "a spot." The neurologist called it "a tumor." Niek was 42 years old, I was 30.

It announced its presence when Niek developed the look of a serial killer, moving his shoulders forward and back again, and uttering non-sense in a strange, sonorous voice. This would last a minute or so, and repeat several times. Afterwards he remembered nothing. One day my brother was there, and observed it. I asked him if what he had just seen was normal. No, it absolutely wasn't. My brother confirmed my suspicions: something was wrong.

When it also came over him at work, Niek agreed to see a physician. That is when they discovered the pea. This was quite a relief. Now we knew that he was experiencing mild epileptic seizures, and we knew what was causing them. And things that have a cause are less frightening. Even though the cause was a brain tumor, we were not unduly worried; the pea was small and it was in a favorable location. It just needed to be monitored.

In the meantime Niek enthusiastically threw himself into an allergy. Not that he did not have one; he had sneezed his way through many summers. When, in 1995, he started blaming the increasingly serious epileptic seizures on the allergy it dawned on me that he was in denial. Because allergies do not cause epilepsy.

Niek's personality was also changing. He gradually withdrew into another world. He had always been a dreamer, but now he was seeing galaxies filled with God, love and eternal bliss. Not all the time, because in addition to feeling euphoric, he was also distrustful, resentful, and distant more and more often. And many creatures had apparently taken up residence in our home. Every now and then he would say something about them. One of them, for example, was a baker's wife who frightened him. Even though he knew it was his imagination, he still put the rusk tin on top of the refrigerator to assuage her. A whirling dervish on the other hand, gave him confidence, as did a snowman that occasionally entered the living room bathing in light and made Niek look up in delight.

While Niek was busy with these houseguests, my work often took me abroad. Our relationship began to suffer under the pressure.

"Going home already?" a colleague asked me one January night in 1996. "Yes, I need to leave early, Niek is in the hospital. He is going to have brain surgery tomorrow, to remove a tumor." When I saw her look of shock I was ashamed. "It isn't that bad," I reassured her. "Well, brain tumor, it's just a small spot. And it is in a very favorable location." The tumor had started to change, the neurologist said, and so it had to come out now.

That night, when I saw that they had automatically put Niek in a single hospital room, it registered that brain surgery, even for a small pea, is a serious matter. Or maybe I hadn't wanted to see it until now. I said goodbye to Niek, tried to reassure him. I was prepared for the very slim chance he would die. What I did not reckon with was the also very slight chance he would become disabled.

Niek was a person who could walk into a bar and within an hour he would be talking to a complete stranger who would entrust him with his most private thoughts and feelings. Usually a woman. Niek had many good women friends. He, on the other hand, rarely shared anything.

He had never told me, for example, that he had been terrified that the operation would leave him disabled. Every time he entered to the hospital for one of his many appointments, the wheelchair entrance caught his eye. Afterwards the surgeon told me that no patient had ever interrogated him so extensively about the risk of becoming disabled as a result of the brain surgery. The chance of this happening was very slim, as the surgeon repeated again after the surgery, looking at Niek in amazement.

The following evening, after Niek's surgery, I visited him in the intensive care unit. He seemed almost conscious and he squeezed my hand as if he was afraid he would die. I saw then that his left side did not move, that half of him was motionless from his arm down to his leg. However, I was more afraid of his death.

The next day the neurosurgeon was pacing around Niek's bed. He was worried and seemed to be upset. The "small pea" turned out to be more like an egg, with small tails. The tumor was gone, but the operation had unexpectedly resulted in a severe brain injury.

When the physician left I sat by Niek's bed. He had always loved reading the Oliver Sacks books, about the brain and how it functions when it is affected. He was unaware that he was now saying something that Sacks described exactly like this: "This morning I thought they had put someone in bed with me, because I felt a strange leg next to me. But it was my own leg." He had not recognized his paralyzed leg as his own. A moment later he wanted to touch me. I didn't have the heart to tell him he was caressing his own left arm.

Niek was confused. I had to explain to him that when it is dark it is night, and when it is light it is day. That we sleep when it is night and that he should not telephone me then. And I wondered what was in store for us if I had to explain something as obvious as this. I knew this was worse than the arm and the leg that did not work anymore.

After one month in hospital, Niek was moved to the rehabilitation center, where he would remain for nine months.

One psychologist at the rehabilitation center frightened Niek, but reassured me. The psychologist tested Niek's remaining intellectual abilities. This was hard on Niek, so he hated the psychologist. I was happy with the psychologist. He determined scientifically what I had known for a long time: not only was Niek paralyzed on the left side, his mind was affected too.

He learned to walk a few steps with his right leg during rehabilitation; his left leg, harnessed in a brace, became like a cane. Getting dressed was impossible, because Niek had no idea of the difference between a trouser leg, a sleeve and a neck opening.

Plus he forgot his left side. Niek was not only paralyzed on the left side, he also denied and ignored all things left. If I told him to look to the left, he would look up. To the ophthalmologist's delight he had a perfect hemianopia, or blindness in half the visual field: the brain processed only the right half of the visual field for both eyes. At dinner he finished only the right half of his plate, because he could not see the left half. However, he quickly worked out that if you turned the plate you would always find seconds. When he tried to read, he only saw the right half of the line. After a while he managed to read simple newspaper headlines and CD titles from the third or fourth word, and he would subsequently guess the first words.

His left arm hung paralyzed and twisted in front of his chest and was constantly in the way. His face was asymmetrical due to the paralysis and now and then spittle would drip from the left corner of his mouth. Niek was no longer aware of space, he lacked all spatial sense, and he bumped into everyone to the left side with of his wheelchair. He was always looking for his things, he lost his way even inside the house and lost himself in the chaos. Time no longer existed, but by surrounding himself with clocks Niek hoped to find some stability.

When I walked into the rehabilitation center I would often find him with a confused, anxious look in his eye, desperately searching for something to hold onto. The brain injury look. As soon as he saw me his face would light up, he would relax and look at me affectionately with a sweet and funny look. He was not the same person I had been with for seven years. Niek was much more affectionate, childlike, sweeter. And a lot less intelligent.

The rehabilitation specialist advised me against bringing Niek home; this would certainly be too burdensome. He suggested sending him to a nursing home. At some point Niek could move from there to a living accommodation for people with brain injury. But Niek clung to me, to Leiden, to our house, and I was very sure about two things. Niek had to come home, or his spirit would be broken. And Niek could not come home, because the rehabilitation specialist was right and it would be too much.

This dilemma was complicated – once he was back home it would be virtually impossible to find assisted-living accommodation for a brain-injured man. In the wait-list battle for scarce spots in assisted-living accommodations, candidates who lived at home usually lost. Patients transferred from hospitals and nursing homes always won. I decided to bring Niek home because of the look in his eye. The brain injury look that calmed down when he saw me. My presence reassured him, and that made me responsible for him.

In the autumn of 1996 Niek came home. From then on, I usually worked at night so I had time during the day for Niek, and for the range of agencies and organizations we now had to deal with. If I was not there and Niek needed help, he could press an alarm button; the emergency switchboard would then phone one of his friends. They all had keys and were ready to pitch in. Which was a good thing, because instead of mild epileptic seizures Niek now had severe seizures. Fortunately he could feel them coming so he was able to quickly press the alarm before the seizure started.

Despite the brain damage, Niek's memory had remained intact. He could learn things by heart and then apply them routinely. I arranged computer lessons for Niek. After several years of practice he was able to send emails and download music. Work was no longer possible; he could not teach anymore. This upset Niek greatly, because he was born to stand in front of a classroom. Niek now spent his days playing CDs and LPs, or videos and DVDs. Sometimes he managed to put together beautiful CDs with music that made all his friends happy. There were other times when he would search for a specific clip from *Absolutely Fabulous* for six hours, even searching for the non-existent B-sides of DVD's and video tapes. When he could not find the clip, he would start over, and repeat the same searches with the same results.

At moments like those, there was no getting through to him. He could not control his attention anymore; if an attempt at something failed, he could go on trying all day. Apparently the ability to draw a line under a "project" is also a brain function that can be surgically removed. At night I would clear away the stacks of LPs, CDs, videos and DVDs around him, and Niek would invariably get angry that he wouldn't be able to find anything. The absence of a sense of time meant that he did not want to go to bed before the middle of the night.

Niek had a lot of fun with the home care people, telling jokes and playing pranks. He continued to make new friends. Even though I had to write a manual to explain some of his sometimes strange reactions, Niek remained sociable and able to sense how people were doing. In this way he was also able to support me. All in all he had visitors at least several times a week.

Niek was not able to go out on his own; as soon as he was out the door he would get lost. Besides, he had scrapped the entire concept of "left." He could not comprehend traffic coming from the left. For a long time I hoped that Niek would one day be able to make a fixed daily trip around the neighborhood with a guide dog and a mobility scooter, so he could get out of the house more. This always proved too ambitious. The risk that he would end up in a ditch was too great. So Niek stayed inside and only went outside with assistance. Once a week someone from home care took Niek into town. He could leave the house and buy things, or borrow CDs at the CD rental service. They always had a stack ready and waiting for him. Sometimes we would go into the woods with friends, or visit rock concerts.

"He'd be better off dead"

In the summer of 1998, two and a half years after Niek's brain was injured, I met one of his friends on the train to Amsterdam. We greeted each other and started talking about Niek. "Wouldn't it have been better if he had died during the operation?" he said. It took me by surprise that a friend of Niek who had gone on holiday with him a few years earlier could say this. I wanted to be honest – hadn't I secretly thought the same thing a few times? "I sometimes thought it would have been easier for me if he had died," I admitted. "Because then I could have said goodbye and moved on. But for him it is a good thing that he is alive. Sometimes he laughs, he loves music." "No, it would have been better if he had died – for him as well," Niek's friend insisted. This statement has haunted me ever since.

Another one of Niek's acquaintances came over for dinner one night. Still wound up from her busy job she said to Niek: "You choose to go on living, so you have no right to whine." Apart from the fact that Niek rarely whined, this remark struck me. It was as if she was saying to Niek: I would understand completely if you ended it. If you don't want to, then you should not talk about your disabilities. And I don't have to sympathize with you. Another remark to haunt me.

Goodbyes

More than four years after Niek sustained his brain injury I decided to leave him. Not leave him permanently, but create some distance. As long as I was around, the health care agencies, family and friends all thought that Niek was being taken care of. Thanks to my industrious management of the whole situation everybody was confident that Niek was in good hands; I was getting compliments left and right for my commitment and loving care. However, to me these compliments were like the bars of my cage. It felt like nobody could imagine the possibility of me breaking down, which actually brought the moment undeniably closer. I was afraid that I would start hitting Niek one day. Leaving was the best option, so when I was offered a job in Berlin I took it. Now I had a deadline: that summer I was going to move to Germany. And everything started shifting: Niek accepted a small apartment near a care home that would receive extra money from the government to take care of him during the night in case of an emergency – the amount of home care was increased considerably – and his family agreed to step up and do more.

Now I could leave. When, after five months of preparation, the moment of having to leave Niek behind arrived, it felt like I was tearing off my own arm. Niek did not blame me for anything. He did cry for two seconds. It was one of the few times in his life that I saw Niek cry.

Four weeks later I came back for a long weekend. That would be the monthly routine from then on. We were both very happy to see each other. The next three days I took care of the paperwork, cleaned, cooked meals for many days ahead, tidied up, and took care of Niek to save on home care. And he played music for me. When I was in Berlin we would talk on the phone every day, officially only at 11:30 pm, so Niek would know it was time to go to bed, but Niek usually found some excuse to call at least twice during the day. Now that I was no longer collapsing under the care, I was able to take Niek on vacation once a year; friends went with us to help carry him when necessary.

The best time started four years later. Niek moved into a wheelchair-accessible ground floor apartment across the street from a nursing home. Before this move he would enjoy some sunshine on his fifth-floor balcony on his own, but now you could find him in his small garden six months of the year. Niek spoke to all passers-by. He saw more people than ever before. Moreover, after much practice Niek managed to get himself to the nursing home across the street in his wheelchair, to get a haircut, or go to physical therapy. For the first time in nine years he could get out of his apartment and go somewhere on his own, even if it was no more than one hundred yards. And if he did fall, wheelchair and all, neighbors were always around to help him. After four years I moved back to the Netherlands from Berlin and I now lived in Amsterdam, half an hour away from him.

It was a timely return, because Niek took a turn for the worse in July 2005. He fell down more often, so often that after a while he was afraid to go to the bathroom or to bed and preferred to stay in his chair all day. The home care people expressed their concern, but I stubbornly continued to reassure everyone, and especially myself. One day Niek confessed he had unsuccessfully tried to put on a shoe for eight hours; it worried him that he had kept on for so long without looking up, without drinking or eating anything. His disabilities became worse. When Niek ate, his head tilted increasingly to the left and his forehead would be in his food. He could no longer bring the fork to his mouth with his right arm; by the end of the month I was feeding him.

One night - my colleagues had sent me home early - I realized that it was time for Niek to go to hospital. We could not go on like this, and our family doctor agreed with me.

Late at night, at the hospital, I betrayed Niek. "What is your relationship to the patient?" the nurse asked. "A friend," I said, not knowing how to define my relationship with Niek to the outside world. "You're not a friend, you are my boyfriend," Niek said sharply. He was right; although Niek was not the same man he was when we were in a relationship, and I'd had a series of affairs in Berlin and Amsterdam, Niek was still the man I felt closest to.

Two days later the whole family gathered in the hospital. The physicians wanted to talk to us, and their lack of urgency told me they had bad news. The tumor had returned, the once little pea now measured six by nine centimeters. An operation was possible, but risky, and would only delay his death. No operation would mean Niek did not have much time left, a few weeks perhaps. By then Niek was unconscious; although we discussed all this at his bedside, he heard nothing.

His brother, sister-in-law and I decided against the operation, because after the first operation Niek said that he never wanted to have another one. After two days he came home, where a hospital bed was placed in the living room. By fighting the fluids surrounding the tumor with medication, he regained consciousness to some degree. Enough for me to tell him what was going on. The first day I told Niek he was going to die. The second day he asked me how much time he had and I told him "not very much." The third day Niek probed deeper: "What did the neurologist say exactly?" I said: "A few weeks." Niek now told me he had suspected for a while that the tumor had returned, because on our vacation earlier that year in the countryside in the eastern part of the Netherlands, the birds had looked at him funny.

Two more times we went to the beach, where Niek, a true descendant of Scheveningen fishermen, belonged. Niek's brother and two friends came along to drag the wheelchair through the sand.

He lived another four months. With friends and family we did most of the care ourselves. The gibberish coming out of Niek's mouth now that the tumor was growing did not change the fact that we continued to understand each other remarkably well. "Here's the fusspot," he cried out merrily when I walked in one time and he, thanks to a higher dose of medicine, briefly felt better. Eventually Niek caught a cold and lost consciousness. The sight of a dying Niek shocked everybody who came to his deathbed. Nevertheless, the atmosphere around him was cheerful and pleasant, like it had always been with Niek. He died on November 28 2005, at home, surrounded by friends.

The ten years that Niek had lived with his injured brain, were heavy, but every bit as valuable as the years before that. That is why I could not get past the remark that Niek would be "better off dead." Where does such a remark about a disabled friend come from?

Niek died a natural death. But could the judgment of a friend that it would have been better if Niek had died rather than survive, disabled, for another ten years, perhaps be traced back to the euthanasia law? One consequence of people being able to speak about their own death and about the question whether death is in some cases preferable to life, is that they may also make the judgment about others – that they are better off dead. Sometimes people say they would rather be dead when they are diagnosed with a particular illness. Could it be that they reason that others who are struck by the same illness would also prefer to be dead? Does the judgment of what one does not want for oneself under any circumstances turn into an opinion about what others should not want? Has our thinking about euthanasia, where people get to decide their own end of life, unintentionally also influenced how we think about other people's lives?

Despair

I also made judgments about Niek's life from time to time. In moments of despair I even wished my disabled partner dead.

When Niek woke up in 1996 after the operation, without the tumor but with disabilities, he pinned his hopes on me. Our bond deepened. The man I had been relying on for seven years was gone. In his place was a sweet, strange younger brother who needed my care. He relied on me. That was beautiful as it was heavy. Beautiful, because never before in my life did I feel this useful, or my mere presence make anyone look so happy. Heavy, because he expected me to take him back to earlier days, back to the times of long walks in the woods, back to the day he walked into the hospital. And I was unable.

At times I didn't want to take care of him at all. When he needed me the most – that is when I sometimes wanted to run. The moment Niek became disabled proved to be an excellent moment for evaluation: Was the relationship really that good? Didn't we have our problems? Didn't I have doubts about us sometimes?

Much as I loved him, from the moment Niek's brain was injured our interests no longer coincided; they were as different as our two futures, as different as what we could do with the rest of our lives. Put more bluntly: I could leave, he could not. Tears filled my eyes when a colleague said: "You can't be expected to give up your whole life for him, can you?" This was exactly the question I was asking myself at that time.

I often had fantasies of escaping in those days. Some were fantasies about death – his, or ours. Niek also talked about death as a way out immediately after the operation.

Because memories are unreliable, I quote from the journal that I kept for a few years since 1996. Reading it again, I see that I mentioned death more often than I can now remember, or even imagine.

On January 30 1996 Niek had been disabled for four days. The realization that his left leg and arm were paralyzed was beginning to set in. He wanted to flee from the hospital, and fought to get out of bed. The fact that half of his body remained motionless despite his efforts was something he was not ready to see. In my journal I wrote: "Niek was defiant all day and reproaches (a good friend) and me that we won't help him get out of bed. 'Look, both my feet are already on the chair, if you help me now I'll be out of bed in no time.' In reality only one leg was on that chair. 'Help me, you coward, you're chicken aren't you'." While Niek was concerned about his left arm and leg being paralyzed, my main fear was that his personality had changed. "An arm, a leg, who cares, as long as Niek stays the same Niek… Last Sunday I thought for a second: if he turns into a vegetable we'll take an overdose together. But of course I won't do that."

At the end of February 1996, after a month in the hospital, Niek was transferred to a rehabilitation center on the coast in Katwijk aan Zee. In

my journal I wrote that day: "I feel like I am taking Niek to an old people's home... Leaving the hospital was difficult too: this is where things
went wrong, a month ago now. Now that we have taken the next step it
seems even more difficult to go back to the time before the operation...
Fighting the tears all day long... Niek was probably experiencing the
same emotions, but he did not express them. He only talked about pain,
hunger, thirst, peeing. I thought – in a moment of selfishness – that it
would have been easier for me to accept Niek dying than this."

March 1996: "I can tell I am desperate by the fact that I tend to see
suicide, together with Niek, as the only way out. But that's impossible,
it's not necessary and I can't do that to (my sister and brother)."

"Niek comes home for the Whitsun weekend. It takes me hours to get
Niek on the toilet chair in the living room, wash and dress him and give
him breakfast. He despairs: 'I wish I had died on the operating table.' I
managed to talk him out of that thought, absolutely the right thing to do,
but sometimes I do think it is easier for a partner to live with the sudden
death of your boyfriend than with his sudden dependence on you."

Niek was coming home for the weekend more often now. On Sunday nights I would take him back to the rehabilitation center in Katwijk
aan Zee. Early June 1996: "Niek told me this weekend that he has a
ghost inside him that forces him to constantly think about ways to end it,
and tells him: 'You don't have the balls anyway', during every therapy
session. Niek felt he was a burden and asked me if I am happy when I
can take him back to Katwijk. I didn't have the heart to say yes, partly
because - and I did tell him this - there is a difference between being a
burden because you need help with the everyday activities or being a
burden because you're a horrible person."

July 1996: "Niek dreamed about driving into the canal and ending it
again, "but I can't do that to you." No, perish the thought, although I too
sometimes see death / his death / our death as the only way out."

In the summer of 1996 Niek was learning to get from his wheelchair
on to the bed or the toilet without help at the rehabilitation center; he

wouldn't be allowed to go home until he could do this. But it was a struggle. I wrote in my journal: "He is suspicious and blames me for telling the staff in Katwijk all the things he is not able to do at home. It's true: Niek can do some transfers on his own. But this morning he positioned the wheelchair completely wrong. When I intervened before he fell, he was furious with me. We have landed in a nightmare and I sometimes – increasingly – see death as the only way out."

Early August the mood lifted a little: "Sometimes it is as if Niek peers through a crack in a coffin. He can see his school, he can see the steps that lead upstairs: he knows what rock concerts are planned, but he can't go there anymore. And for the last six months we have been working hard to widen the crack in the coffin. Because it definitely was a coffin that Niek ended up in, but as it turned out: it was not meant for him yet. Niek is alive, and he seems to be climbing out, especially now that he is learning how to walk again."

When Niek was coming home, we were both happy. With his disabilities, however, the challenge of everyday life almost proved too much. Home care services and friends were helping out, and Niek was making the biggest effort of all. Still, we could barely cope. After two years I started investigating the possibility of placing Niek in a care home. This turned out to be far from simple – it could take years. Every now and then I contemplated fleeing the situation, just to force the authorities to find a place in an institution for Niek.

September 1998: "I just went into a state of panic. Niek was also extremely agitated and clearly has not been getting enough rest these last days… I thought about writing a letter to all our friends: 'Dear friends, faced with the choice between hanging myself and running away, I have opted for the latter. I am not telling you where I am going and I am never coming back. Please take good care of Niek.' It's like my thoughts are getting the better of me." However, the panic subsided quickly: "Now that I am by myself for a while I am calming down. I will take good care of Niek, one way or another, and make him understand it is a good thing that he is alive."

Niek, in the meantime, would take special delight when he talked about the old days. "Last Sunday morning Niek was feeling sad, he had had another bad night and was restless... I sat on the edge of his bed and put his head in my lap and stroked his hair. He looked at me, so sad and so happy that I did that, he surrendered to me briefly and let me comfort him. He has been feeling nostalgic lately, he said. I agree. His eyes sparkle only when he talks about the past... It's strange, because I am living completely in the future and I can't wait for the second half of my life to begin, when I will be on my own again."

Informal Caregivers

The deterioration of someone you care about confronts you with your own shortcomings, because this is something you can't fix. Because brain damage causes changes in an individual's personality, you need to mourn the loss of the person who is no longer there. Yet because he still is there and needs your care, you can't mourn. What is more, you don't have the time. Of course you will think of death as being a solution in dark or rebellious moments; your death or the death of the other person; the person that you love but who now needs your care.

But that is all it should be, I think. An impulse. When I realized the fundamental changes in Niek, so fundamental that I did think once or twice that he would be better off dead, I was shocked. What right did I have to think this?

Thoughts about the death of the person you are taking care of are an indication it is time to turn the love down a bit, to take some distance from the suffering the other person is going through. Love is a beautiful thing, but if you let it lead you into the dumps as well, then you are no good to the other person. It does not help the other person if the people who love him start doubting whether his life still has meaning, especially now that he needs them so badly. If you do, it is better to leave the caring to someone else, limit your love to taking care of the paperwork or clearing out the closets. Do not start contemplating the other person's death as a solution.

I never thought of death as a way out after Niek got his own place in 2000, under the protection of the nursing home and with plenty of home care. I was there for him when we talked on the phone (several times a day), when I went to visit him (one long weekend every month) and when I organized a vacation for him (two weeks a year), but the rest of the time I had my own life in Berlin. After a while Niek realized that I kept coming back and I did not give up on him. At least not completely.

Other people who have a wife or husband with brain damage turn out, like myself, to have thought about death as a way out. When I attend a meeting of a patient association for people with non-congenital brain damage, I get to know a group of partners there. We can almost read each other's minds, regardless of whether we have a wife with pre-eclampsia, a husband who was in a car accident or a partner with a brain tumor. Someone asks me if I had ever secretly thought it would be better if Niek had died. "Yes, at times," I answer, surprised at the poignant question, and he grins, because he knew; he had thought the same about his severely disabled wife.

Parents of a seriously ill or disabled baby also sometimes feel the urge to run. Just like I started doubting my relationship with Niek at the moment he became disabled, parents of a disabled child demonstrate similar escape behavior in a different way. Pediatrician Van Bruggen on the subject: "The child you expected did not come. Your dreams are not fulfilled. Yet then there is this other child, the child you did not expect... The child puts a claim on the parents: I belong to you. A period of strong ambivalence in the relationship between parents and child follows. Many parents have a flight response. They want their child to be dead. Very few of them have the courage to let these wishes penetrate their consciousness or express them."[144]

Caring for a seriously ill or disabled person can be tough and death may look like a way out. But does it help informal caregivers when the

---

144   G. van Bruggen, quoted in P.J. Lieverse et al., *Dood gewoon? Perspectieven op 35 jaar euthanasie in Nederland*, Amsterdam, Buijten en Schipperheijn, 2005, p. 45 [Dead simple? Perspectives on 35 years of euthanasia in the Netherlands]

death of the person they take care of actually becomes an option? Does it help people in a crisis to have more options to choose from? Does it help when the one you take care of dies, maybe after you have pleaded to discontinue medical treatment? And are you, being the one who takes care of the person, the right person to make such decisions?

People who provide care are not selfless saints; I know I wasn't. People who care are not the person they take care of; the solidarity that moves you to take care of another person does not mean you are in the same situation. On the contrary, it is exactly because informal caregivers take care of someone that their interests are not the same as those of the person being taken care of.

For all the discussion in the Netherlands about end-of-life decisions for individuals who are unable to make these decisions for themselves, this difference between the caregiver and the patient is too easily overlooked. It is all very well to say that if the patient is no longer able to make his own decisions, his family and partner have the right to do it for him. Yet however much you love a person, it does not mean that you are also the right person to make decisions, in his place, in his interest, about his life. The question whether to treat, abstain from treatment or terminate the life of the person you take care of is difficult to decide for you as the caregiver without your own interests becoming mixed up with the interests of the person you take care of. Because informal caregivers are also stakeholders they are not in a position to make decisions about the life or death of the person they take care of. Their love for the person they take care of does not alter that fact; not when caring becomes difficult and desperation hits, that is.

It would be a good thing to place limits on the decisions that informal family caregivers are allowed to make. If the caregiving family collapses under the responsibilities of care, the life of the person they are making decisions for must still be protected. In the case of a child with multiple disabilities who contracts pneumonia, a course of antibiotics is not burdensome, and might add years to his life. It would be reasonable to deny the baby's parents the power to refuse that treatment.

The reality is that those limits have been shifting over the past four decades. In the Netherlands, no limits have been applied to the discussions of the many questions at the start and the end of life, so the limits to practice have been blurred or erased. This need not be a problem when you have to make a decision, without haste and well considered. Yet it can be a problem if you have to reach a decision when you are totally overburdened.

Even when termination of life or abstaining from medical treatment is not being considered for a particular patient, the society continues to debate the value of a life with disability or illness. The very openness with which these things are discussed affects the relationship between the disabled person and the people around him. If you, as the caregiver, take care of a person day in and day out, it makes a difference what the people around think. It makes a difference whether they agree that there is no alternative, or whether they think, and perhaps even say: this isn't necessary, is it?

Termination of life or abstaining from treatment in the case of severely disabled or ill babies, children and adults, euthanasia in elderly people with dementia and assisted suicide for psychiatric patients – all of these things unavoidably affect the relationship between people with these severe conditions and their caregivers.

To deny this is to create a new taboo.

A Physician's Judgment

Family and friends are not the only people whose decisions about ill and disabled persons may reflect their own ideas more than the ideas of the people they are judging. Even physicians, consciously or subconsciously, allow their decision about patients to be influenced by personal views of what makes life valuable and under which circumstances a person is better off dead. Sometimes a physician assesses the life of a seriously ill or disabled patient in a way that reveals the view of life of the physician in question.

Here is an example that played out in the newspaper *de Volkskrant* in 2008. When the NVVE insisted that euthanasia should be more accessible for people with dementia, columnist Aleid Truijens countered with a warning about the dangers of this move.

Rob Jonquière, a physician and the director of euthanasia association NVVE, responded to Truijens. Death is postponed thanks to medical intervention and societal progress, Jonquière wrote. "The empowered person today is not always served by this postponement, especially if he feels it means a goodbye without dignity. In the Netherlands this person can and may in many cases request a dignified end of life. I consider this an achievement of our society. When they do not get the end of life that they want, people demand that the debate is continued. Truijens has the right to choose to risk walking around like a zombie in a dirty diaper at some point in her life. Just as she has the right to receive optimal care, which would then give her the type of death she chooses. Are we allowed to make a different choice?"

In a liberal tone, the letter launches with the principles of self-determination of the NVVE. Jonquière presented "the empowered person today," who wants a "dignified end of life." In "our society" he would have this choice. This is the reassuring, broadminded language of the liberals, the language of self-determination.

Jonquière promptly moved from self-determination to severe judgment: the person living with dementia is "a zombie in a dirty diaper." In one and the same paragraph, Jonquière's commitment to a self-determined 'dignified' death immediately escalated into the judgment that a natural death is an undignified death, like a "zombie in a dirty diaper." In an interview with *NRC Handelsblad* two weeks earlier, the NVVE director had referred to people with Alzheimer's disease who had chosen a natural death as "wasting away like zombies in dirty diapers."[145] Jonquière's rhetoric about 'self-determination' and a "dignified end of life" led him to judge other people in harsh words.

---

145 Elsbeth Etty, De stelling van Rob Jonquière: aanvaard alle consequenties van een waardig einde [The position of Rob Jonquière: accept all consequences of a dignified end, *NRC Handelsblad*, April 26 2008

Not all physicians are as outspoken. On the contrary, some physicians have discerned that their influence on a patient can be significant. When a patient who is ill but of sound mind asks his physician for euthanasia, it appears to be on their own initiative. Physician Groen-Evers has noticed that the demand for euthanasia depends on whether or not she raised the subject. In the past, says Groen-Evers in an interview with reporter Margriet Oostveen in *NRC Handelsblad*, when conversing with a terminal patient for whom no further treatment option was available, she felt obliged to speak of 'euthanasia'. "Otherwise people would be too shy to discuss it, I thought. And nine times out of ten the patient would return with a request for euthanasia." Ever since she started investigating palliative care, she consciously avoids using the E-word. "And what do you know: almost no one asks for it anymore!" Could that be because patients are simply afraid to ask if she does not mention the word? "No, it really wasn't necessary anymore. And patients are influenced much more than physicians realize. If you mention euthanasia, they will ask for it. If you mention palliative care, then that is what they choose."[146] Apparently man is not the autonomous, self-determining being after all; he lets his physician influence him.

The role of the physician is even more significant when considering termination of life in incompetent patients, such as babies. The arguments justifying termination of the life of an incompetent patient appear to follow those justifying euthanasia. The argument articulated by the Supreme Court to justify euthanasia in the 1980s addressed one key element: the dilemma facing the physician. On the one hand, the physician is obligated to prevent suffering by agreeing to the patient's request for euthanasia. On the other hand, the physician must respect the life of the patient. In specific situations, the physician may resolve the dilemma by responding to the request of his patient and ending his life.

In the case of incompetent patients who suffer severely, physicians can find themselves in a similar dilemma. In this case, some physicians argue, the dilemma can be resolved by considering the termination of

---

146 Margriet Oostveen, Spijt. Voorvechters van de euthanasiepraktijk bezinnen zich [Regret. Proponents reflecting on the euthanasia practice], *NRC Handelsblad*, November 10 2001

life as the lesser of two evils. In two decisions the courts have accepted this argument. In this situation a physician may appeal to *force majeure*: 'in a situation of necessity', the physician is not liable to punishment.[147]

However, these two situations are not the same. In the case of euthanasia, the patient asks for something. The physician's dilemma is the duty of following the patient's request versus the duty not to kill. Yet when the life of an incompetent individual is terminated, the patient has not asked for anything. The role of the physician is therefore much larger, jurist Jo Dorscheidt observes. It is the physician who perceives the conflict between his duty to prevent suffering and his duty not to kill. "The urge to choose in this dilemma basically starts with and exists inside the physician. The actual initiative for termination of life originates in him. By giving in to this pressure the physician can in some cases also be blamed for having put himself in the situation of necessity presented by him," Dorscheidt writes.[148]

In short: termination of the lives of people who cannot make this decision themselves is about the physician, to a greater degree than in the case of euthanasia. The physician feels he is faced with a dilemma because his patient is suffering. The physician considers ending the patient's life the best way to resolve his dilemma. If there are parents in the picture, for example because it concerns a newborn, their consent is desired, but the initiative still rests with the physician. In the Groningen Protocol for termination of life in newborns, the parents' consent is mandatory, but it is the physician who takes the initiative.[149] This is the opposite of euthanasia: the patient takes the initiative and the physician consents.

The heated discussions among physicians described in chapter three about the point or pointlessness of terminating the lives of babies born with spina bifida indicate how differently physicians sometimes think

---

147 See chapter 4 on the *Kadijk* and *Prins* cases

148 Dorscheidt, op. cit., p. 93

149 See also Theo Boer, Recurring Themes in the Debate about Euthanasia and Assisted Suicide, *Journal of Religious Ethics*, 35, 3 (2007), p. 544

about the subject. Physicians are people, with their own ideas about life and death. The fact that the life of newborns with spina bifida is sometimes ended in one Dutch hospital, and this never happens in another, demonstrates just how much physicians' opinions can differ.

Ethicist Hans Reinders describes how the physicians' views on what makes life valuable may influence how they deal with their patients. Physicians and caregivers might believe that the valuable life consists in each individual developing into something greater. Writing about the care of people with mental disabilities, Reinders noted the tendency of caregivers to want these dependent individuals to develop, even the severely handicapped ones.[150] If caregivers apply this way of thinking, it implies that the treatment must help the disabled individual improve. When this proves impossible, medical staff are confronted with their own limits. This is uncomfortable. Reinders quotes the German remedial educationalist Emil Kolb, who describes this phenomenon: "When there is nothing more to examine or to do, the researchers and doers are confronted with the possible futility of their own actions. And this must not be allowed to happen!" Physicians cannot allow the disabled individual to simply be; they must help him to develop. Emil Kolb summarizes this belief "What cannot become something, must be nothing."

How a physician views his own life must be important, says Reinders, because this view affects the physician's ideas on the value of a dependent disabled life. People who consider their own development and independence to be important and who see themselves as the author, creator of their own life story, filled with choices and possibilities, will have a problem with individuals who are dependent on other people and experience no development at all. "From the perspective of people who view their own existence as a project of which they themselves… are the author, a severely disabled life must inevitably seem completely

---

150 Hans Reinders, "Wat niets kan worden, stelt niets voor." Mensen met een ernstige verstandelijke handicap in het licht van de hedendaagse gezondheidsethiek. Een kritische uiteenzetting. Inaugurele rede, Amsterdam, VU, Amersfoort, 's Heeren Loo, 1996 ["If it cannot become something, it is nothing." People with a severe mental handicap in the perspective of current health ethics]

pointless. A condition that appears to them like death, even if it does not coincide with it."[151]

On the other hand, people who believe that we are not isolated individuals, that we are all dependent on other human beings, will have less trouble dealing with a person who is much more dependent on others. People whose ideals are more grounded than 'self-fulfillment' will find it easier to deal with individuals whose disability or illness make self-fulfillment irrelevant.

Self-development is a beautiful, humanistic ideal, so it seems a good thing when a physician considers development a life goal. Yet such a lofty ideal can also lead the physician to a sense of self-importance that is hostile to people who have diminished possibilities for self-fulfillment. Such people cannot live up to what, according to the physician, makes life meaningful.

An Ethicist's Judgment

Few public figures illustrate how an individual's personal philosophy can lead to judgments about other people better than Heleen Dupuis. Always popular in the media, this Dutch ethicist and politician has managed to draw more attention to herself over the past thirty years than perhaps any other person in the medical-ethical debate. A theologian by profession, Dupuis received her PhD degree in 1976 with a thesis on a medical-ethical subject; she has been active in this field ever since, holding positions on numerous committees. In the decisive period 1981 to 1985, the years of the final breakthrough of euthanasia in the Netherlands, Dupuis was the president of the NVVE. Since 1999 she has been a senator for the right-wing liberal party VVD. (In North America, this party might be called libertarian)

During her career, Dupuis has described many cases of severely ill or disabled individuals. Despite the differences between these cases, and despite her emphasis on the need to judge each case on its own merits, she usually presents the same solution: let the individual die.

---

151 Reinders, op. cit, p. 43

If necessary, cause him to die. For the dilemmas that she described, Dupuis consistently offers death as best way out. When one individual's life brings too little joy and too much suffering, either to the individual in question or those around him, it is better if that person dies.

At the root of Dupuis' convictions are her ideas of what makes human life valuable. In 1994 she wrote: "The life of a person derives its value above all from the fact that the individual vehicle of this life is aware of this value. The prohibition to kill or let die (in a medical context) therefore relates first of all to the life that is appreciated by the person in question."[152] What exactly does it say here? It says that aware life is worthy of protection. Yet if you are not aware of the value of your life due to illness or disability, then you do not meet the ideals of being human applied by Dupuis. In this case the social prohibitions on killing you or letting you die apply to a lesser degree.

Dupuis calls on physicians to make up their own minds: don't hide behind rules about the sanctity of human life. There are circumstances, according to Dupuis, in which the judgment of the physician holds more weight than what the patient has to say. If, for example, a person draws up an advance directive in which he specifically states that he wants medical treatment in case he falls into a permanent coma, the physician can, if Dupuis has her way, disregard the directive. "There may be situations in which letting a coma patient die is the most adequate expression of respect for his person and his dignity."[153]

The physician's philosophy of life thus becomes more important than the self-determination of the patient. Dupuis' thinking has very little to do with self-determination. In some circumstances, she says, physicians should have the courage to reflect, the courage to decide, and the courage to let their patient die or actively end his life. These circumstances often involve incompetent patients, for example affected babies or mentally disabled individuals who are unable to make their

---

152 Heleen M. Dupuis, Wel of niet behandelen? Baat het niet, dan schaadt het wél, Baarn, Ambo, 1994, p. 144-145 [Treat or not treat? It does hurt to try]

153 Op. cit., p. 146-147

own decisions. A physician should then have the courage to abstain from treatment or choose to terminate the life in question. The essential decision is the interest of the incompetent, the disabled or the ill individual: the physician decides in their interest. Dupuis helps the physician come to his decision.

For a person who claims to look at the interest of the ill or disabled patient, Dupuis pays remarkably little attention to ill or disabled *people*. Analyzing her words it is clear that she speaks to healthy people in general and healthy physicians in particular.

This is what Dupuis writes about a nursing home: "A room full of lifeless old people, no joy in life, almost totally unaware, shadows of their former selves: the prospect of living out your last days there is not an appealing one."[154] This text is addressed to us, the healthy people. We imagine what Dupuis describes. We see Dupuis' image of those old people in our mind's eye. However, this is not about them, about the people whose reality is life in the nursing home. The old people who live there are just objects in her argument. Dupuis refers to the nursing home as "a prospect that is not an appealing one." She speaks only to the people for whom the prospect of this nursing home is a worst-case scenario. Healthy people take center stage. They bring with them, like props, their opinions about the old, ill, and disabled at whom they are looking.

This is also very clear in a 1992 Dupuis' lecture to the feminist magazine *Opzij*. The title of the lecture: "The sanctity of life. The outrage of Heleen Dupuis."[155] The ethicist outlined several examples of disabled life that exist by virtue of modern medicine. Babies who would have died of their illnesses yesterday are saved today. The consequences, according to Dupuis, are horrible: "people survive, sometimes all the way up to their extra disabled old age; a hopeless life, in an institution, plagued by many afflictions, sometimes as a vegetable, sometimes – perhaps worst of all – mentally healthy but with a pitifully poorly func-

---

154 Heleen Dupuis, *Op het scherp van de snede*, p. 161 [At daggers drawn]

155 Heleen Dupuis, De heiligheid van het leven. De woede van Heleen Dupuis, Opzijlezing, in: *Opzij*, juni 1992, p. 46-51 [The sanctity of life. The outrage of Heleen Dupuis]

tioning body." That is why Heleen Dupuis is outraged. In one sentence, she lumps together different forms of disabled life. Whether the person referred to is a "vegetable," or a mentally healthy person with a "pitifully poorly functioning body": in both cases their lives are horrible and would have been better prevented. The second situation, the person with the "pitifully poorly functioning body" who is "mentally healthy" is able to speak about the point or pointlessness of his life. But Dupuis does not ask. Dupuis judges that this disabled person should not have received medical treatment, and should have died.

The philosopher Gerard de Vries analyzed this speech by Heleen Dupuis as if it were a play.[156] On stage is the main character of the play, the ethicist herself. The main character likes to engage in discussion with physicians; they have important roles with much text in Dupuis' play. "The other players on stage have less pronounced profiles." The patients and their families remain virtually invisible. "Finally, the parents of a severely disabled child and patients such as elderly people with dementia play a very small part in the text. Contrary to the physicians mentioned before, none of these actors have any lines… In this play they all have walk-on parts."

The play revolves around the ethicist. Major supporting roles are granted to the physicians she addresses. By speaking to the physicians in this way, the main character shows just how courageous she is. She is not afraid to break taboos. She is not afraid to raise difficult issues. She dares to go out on a limb. She dares to induce physicians to make up their own minds instead of blindly obeying obsolete rules and regulations. The other people - the ill and disabled persons - are mere bit players in the argument.

But the main character's argument affects the lives of those bit players: they are better off dead. In their own interest, of course, and in the interest of their families. Yet neither patient nor family rises above the

---

156 Gerard de Vries, *Gerede twijfel. Over de rol van de medische ethiek in Nederland*, Amsterdam, De Balie, 1993 [Reasonable doubt. About the role of medical ethics in the Netherlands]

status of bit player. Dupuis' point is that the physician must have the courage to make life-or-death decisions about his patients. He should not hide behind rules concerning the sanctity of life. "Perhaps the main objection to the absolute application of the principles 'respect for life' and 'sanctity of life' is that it relieves the physician of the obligation to decide the best course of action in each situation. The more rigid the norm, the less the need to think," she writes.[157] Heleen Dupuis promotes the view that the physicians should claim the ethical space they need to make judgments about their own patients based on their own beliefs and ideas.

Society

The liberal politician fights the notion that all human life is sacred. This belief may originate in Christianity, but many non-Christians also deem human life sacrosanct, and many non-Christians endorse the human rights that safeguard it. At most they will prefer to speak of the 'inviolability of life' instead of using the more Christian-sounding 'sanctity of life'. This is not a dispute between Christians and non-Christians. This is a dispute between one group of people who hold that all humans have the same rights, and another group of people who hold that it is acceptable to draw a line between inviolable humans and other humans .

Giving a woman equal rights means persevering with principle, even when the woman is on her deathbed, or is no longer conscious, or is a newborn, or is severely disabled, or is elderly, or fails to live up to the ideal image of humanity in some other way. The alternative for this equality is that we draw a line somewhere – a line that separates those human lives worthy of protection from other human lives not worthy of protection.

The latter project has been attempted often. In the past it was common to kill children born with abnormalities. Hugo Grotius, the seventeenth century jurist, wrote that to be regarded as *menschen*, as human beings, bodies must be fit to have souls. Babies born with deformities – *monstra* – are not considered to be human beings, and they

---

157 Dupuis (1994), op. cit., p. 31

are generally suffocated immediately[158]. Grotius distinguished between *menschen*, who lived, and *monstra* that were suffocated.

Similar dichotomies that draw a line between inviolable and violable life are still being formulated today. In the 1970s, when the Netherlands started taking the lead in the euthanasia debate, theologian P.J. Roscam Abbing introduces a distinction between "human life" and "physical life." He claimed that termination of the latter is allowed in specific situations.[159] Also in the 1970s the Dutch Health Council's *Committee on Health Ethics and Health Law* proposed the distinction between "bio-somatic life" and "human life." All life is bio-somatic, but when bio-somatic life is not human, medical treatment is not necessary. Bio-somatic life that is "permanently excluded from interpersonal contact and communication with the world" need not be saved by medical treatment.[160]

The boundary is being investigated outside the Netherlands as well. Michael Tooley makes a distinction between "human being" and "person." Not every human being is a person: "Something is a person if and only if it is a continuing subject of experiences and other mental states that can envisage a future for itself and that can have desires about its own future states."[161] This definition of "person" excludes all newborns up to the age of three months; they are "human beings" but not yet "persons." Their lives, according to Tooley, are not yet worthy of protection.

H. Tristam Engelhardt uses a more subtle distinction. He distinguishes "moral persons" who are competent, "social persons" who despite

---

158 In Grotius' own words: "Voor gheboren menschen houd men alleen zodanighen, die 't lichaem hebben bequaem om een redelicke ziele te vatten. Andere wanschapene gheboorten houd men voor geen menschen, maar veel eer is men in deze landen ghewoon de selve terstond te smooren." Groot, H. de, Inleiding tot de Hollandsche Rechtsgeleerdheid. Leiden 1965, quoted in: Van den Boer-van den Berg, op. cit., p. 75

159 P.J. Roscam Abbing, *Toegenomen verantwoordelijkheid. Veranderende ethiek rond euthanasie, eugenetiek en moderne biologie*, Nijkerk, Callenbach, 1972 [Increased responsibility. Changing ethics regarding euthanasia, eugenics and modern biology]

160 Advies inzake euthanasie bij pasgeborenen. Interimadvies, uitgebracht door de Commissie Medische Ethiek van de Gezondheidsraad, Rijswijk, 1975, quoted in: J. Stolk (ed.), Gebroken wereld. Zwakzinnigenzorg en de vraag naar euthanasie, Kampen, Kok, 1988, p. 13 [Interim advice on euthanasia in newborns.]

161 In: Michael Tooley, *Abortion and infanticide*, Oxford, Clarendon Press, 1983

being incompetent are loved by their environment, and people with no rights. The latter group consists of individuals who are incompetent and not loved by anyone.[162]

The best-known proponents of distinguishing between lives that may be violated, and lives that may not, are Peter Singer and Helga Kuhse. These two Australians, whom Heleen Dupuis refers to in her books, feel it is unreasonable to call the life of a human being inviolable simply because he is part of the human race. The most severely handicapped baby has less consciousness than a pig, cow or chicken. The doctrine of the sanctity of life has never stopped man from killing pigs, cows or chickens. Singer and Kuhse conclude that man is therefore also allowed to kill severely disabled babies. Those who do not agree with them are guilty of discrimination against animals that are more conscious than severely handicapped babies.[163]

The Ideal And Death

The key ultimately lies in ideas, in particular our own ideas about ourselves, our notion of 'humankind'. The more our ideas about ourselves conform to the ideal human being who confidently takes charge of his life, the higher the risk that we will leave by the wayside those people who don't live up this ideal. It is precisely the lofty, positive-sounding ideals about mankind that pose a threat to people who are unable to approximate them.

"An (intellectual) elite defines the personhood of individuals based on its own utilitarian, hedonistic principles and subsequently attaches rights, status and worthiness of protection, that are withheld from others. And so one man's luck is another man's death sentence," J. Stolk wrote in a book about the mentally handicapped.[164]

---

162 Quoted in: Margo Trappenburg, op. cit., p. 186

163 Helga Kuhse and Peter Singer, *Should the Baby Live? The Problem of Handicapped Infants*, Oxford, New York, Melbourne, Oxford University Press, 1985, p. 122

164 J. Stolk (ed.), *Gebroken wereld. Zwakzinnigenzorg en de vraag naar euthanasie*, Kok, Kampen, 1988, p. 35 [Broken world. Care of the mentally handicapped and the demand for euthanasia]

Is the Netherlands such a horrible place to live for people who are severely ill or disabled? Not at all. Largely financed by the state, the care of the handicapped is more generous than in many other affluent countries.

It is true that the goal of the care seems to be to activate people so they can participate in society as much as possible. The image of the good life is that people are maximally independent, and this also applies to those who are ill or handicapped. Many people who are ill or disabled have no problems meeting this ideal, especially with the development of extensive provisions in the Netherlands to enable people to live at home for as long as possible.

But the lofty ideals, the attempts to make every individual with an illness or disability meet the ideal image of humanity, also have a dark side. Individuals who, despite the care and good intentions, prove unable to move up to the desired level of independence, communication, development, who stay dependent, unable to do anything, unable to become anything and also incapable of sociable communication, can be expelled from the human family. People need to function independently to the highest possible degree; those who need help can get help, but if this does not produce the desired results, for example because an individual has the mental capacity of a one-year-old, then we do not resuscitate him, then we abstain from providing antibiotics when they are needed, because we argue that death is the best option for this person.

This is the paradox of the high-quality care in the Netherlands: we have such lofty ideals about being human that we are dissatisfied when a person does not meet those ideals despite our best care. In this way an idealistic image of humankind, good care and a medical system that threatens people can coexist together.

CONTEXT: *"She asked 'Do I still have quality of life?' "*

One parents' night at her daughter's school a woman approached Clare Wesselius. "Your husband tells me you need mechanical ventilation during the night. Do you feel you still have quality of life?"

Clare Wesselius relates she was taken aback by this remark, made by a woman she did not know. "I was completely overwhelmed. I went on the defensive, I said: "I can still do this, I still like that." And the rest of the evening I was so angry because I had defended myself and had not been able to put her in her place." Looking back Clare Wesselius feels she should have gotten angry. She felt threatened by the remark about her quality of life.

"Some people can't see beyond my wheelchair. It's impossible to get through to them. When you are healthy you can't imagine that the kind of life I have can also be fun and significant. I experience my life in a totally different way than other people see me. I experience myself as a regular person who undertakes, organizes all kinds of things. I want people to accept me as I am. I may have a disease, but I am not a disease."[165]

---

165 Clare Wesselius died on September 2 2011.

Chapter 9

A Plea For Equanimity

Blurred Boundaries

Shocked by the statement "He would have been better off dead" about someone I loved, I analyzed the arguments that can lead to this judgment. The dilemmas that cause people to make this judgment are real, the tragedies are not fictional.

However, the boundaries of what is acceptable have become unclear. The openness that has existed since 1970 in the Dutch debate about death, initially led to entreaties to allow or cause people with very serious afflictions to die 'in their own interest', which is not always the same as 'at their own request'. In the 1980s the debate took a more liberal turn: at that point, self-determination was pursued. That focused the debate on people who are in full possession of their faculties and wish to decide their own life and death. These are the years in which euthanasia actually broke through previous limits in the Netherlands, allowing a person to request his own death if he was suffering severely.

But this also created confusion that continues to this day. People have the right to request to die, but they do not have the right to force a physician to actually deliver death to them. Contrary to what many people think, the Dutch euthanasia law is not based on self-determination – it is based on the physician's judgment of pity. This causes friction between patients and physicians. The request by the person who wants to die is an important precondition, but it is not the essential justification for euthanasia. The key is that in the justice system and the law, the physician is permitted to end the life of a patient, if the physician judges that the patient is undergoing 'hopeless and unbearable suffering'.

Because such 'hopeless and unbearable suffering' was not limited to people who were able to make their own decisions, termination of life without request was proposed before very long. In the 1990s physicians debated the question whether the lives of incompetent patients could be terminated if their suffering was hopeless and unbearable. Babies and people with dementia were especially considered for termination. The reports written by physicians on the subject demonstrated differences of opinion among the medical professionals. Furthermore, while the reports were not always characterized by logic, they did have far-reaching consequences in the courtroom.

The concept of 'hopeless and unbearable suffering' has proven to be vague. Those who believe that the deciding factor is actual pain are mistaken. Some physicians feel that a baby 'suffers hopelessly and unbearably' if it can be predicted that his disabilities will limit his functioning in the future. Other physicians have a more limited definition of 'hopeless and unbearable suffering' in babies: they feel that at the very least there must be suffering at this moment. Such differences of opinion have had consequences in the Netherlands: it matters in which hospital a disabled baby is born.

The text of the Dutch euthanasia law addresses only euthanasia on request. Each year, however, there are also between 270 and 1000 cases of euthanasia *without* request. This reality contradicts the law. It also contradicts the claims of the euthanasia advocates. In the eighties, they were adamant that termination of life would only be permissible on request; otherwise, it would be considered murder. The Dutch position has shifted since then. Sometimes it is judged that 'in their own interest', incompetent people are better off dead. After physicians have passed that judgment, their lives may actually be terminated – 'in their interest', of course.

This situation was not brought about by Parliament. Physicians formulated the reports on the permissibility of euthanasia without request. Only after these reports were published did the courts follow the physicians. Consider a person whose life is ended without his own request. Are his human rights being respected? That question was never answered in the Netherlands.

Ending a person's life to limit his suffering springs from pity, or, (for those who feel the term "pity" is too old-fashioned) from compassion. Pity is the epitome of paternalism. In the Dutch practice of termination of life without request, self-determination is not a significant factor.

More common – and less controversial – than termination without request is abstaining from life-prolonging treatment. When a physician, based on his professional knowledge, judges a treatment to be futile, he will abstain from it. The debate on such decisions shows that the situation is not always clear-cut. In some cases we must ask: Did the physician abstain from treatment because it was medically futile? Or was treatment discontinued because the life of the patient was judged to be pointless? These are two very different issues. If, for example, a relatively light treatment is not provided merely because the patient is severely disabled, then the decision-maker apparently feels that the patient is better off dead. In the Netherlands, for example, seriously disabled individuals with easily-treated infections are sometimes not provided antibiotics, at the request of the families who feel it is pointless.

The judgment that another person is better off dead begs questions about the person who makes the decision. Does a physician base his judgment on medical facts? Or does he rely upon his own ideas about what makes life worthwhile? A physician with high ideals about human life might question the value of the life of an individual who cannot meet these ideals, due to illness or disability.

When you become responsible for the care of a partner or relative, your interests as a caregiver do not coincide with the interests of the person you are caring for. As a loved one, you may be distressed, you may be desperate. And yet, in the law, in legal precedents and in medical judgment, you have the right to make the decision for the person who is unable to do so himself. The Dutch law puts almost no limits on decisions like these, even when they concern the life and death of another person.

If we have to decide for others, the dilemmas in healthcare will always remain impossible choices. What remains is gray areas, and *force majeure*. All of our efforts of the past forty years to resolve them through medical-ethical debates have resulted in more confusion than anything else. The problem with medical ethics is its core belief that if we weigh up pros and cons we can find a solution to every medical dilemma. The dilemmas in neonatology are tragedies that have no real solution, states philosopher Gerard de Vries. "Contrary to what medical-ethical tradition suggests... these are not situations that can be 'resolved' by listing the interests, rights, duties or preferences at issue, after which a well-founded, balanced decision can be made and the case is closed. It is not a matter of choosing between different types of insurance that all have their own premiums and proceeds. If you are confronted with a tragedy, you soon run into the limits of your language." [166]

Philosopher Hub Zwart also draws attention to the tendency in medical ethics to approach these dilemmas by weighing one person's interests against others. Using this method, finding the way out of our dilemmas becomes a matter of determining how much interest an individual still has in his own life. Yet not everything can be calculated, controlled and solved. Hub Zwart therefore advocates ethical conflict: "The point is to bring out the inconsistencies and investigate them in detail, so that all parties involved move towards the conflict together. An ethical approach to problematical moral situations looks for the conflict." Medical practice in the Netherlands, cautions Zwart, does the opposite: the conflict is avoided and ethics is used only to justify decisions after they have been made. "By the time the medical-ethical committee takes

---

[166] Gerard de Vries, *Gerede twijfel. Over de rol van de medische ethiek in Nederland*, Amsterdam, De Balie, 1993 [Reasonable doubt. About the role of medical ethics in the Netherlands]

the floor, the agenda is often already fixed." [167]

The openness of the Dutch medical-ethical debate has been much praised. It is true that openness may be the beginning of a solution, but only if the outcome is not a foregone conclusion. It should not be the case that everything that is made discussible today, is permitted tomorrow. For in an open debate you can also discuss options only to conclude that it is best to discard them. If the debate in the Netherlands is as open as the Dutch often claim, then it must be possible to call for restraint, prudence and conservatism when the subject is other people's lives.

In my case, the confrontation with my partner's disabilities and other people's reactions caused me to change my thinking. From a Dutchman who, like most Dutch people, regarded euthanasia as a symbol of Dutch progressiveness, I have changed into a person who is more reserved on the subject.

Let the advocates of euthanasia in countries where it is not yet legal learn from the Dutch example. They should ask themselves what should be the most important reason for euthanasia: self-determination or compassion. If they choose self-determination, then they face the question how they think they can prevent their country going down the same path as the Netherlands once euthanasia is allowed.

Ever since they have been allowed to decide for themselves, people in the Netherlands have also started judging other people's lives. What started as self-determination has ended in paternalism towards people who are unable to make their own decisions. This scenario can unfold anywhere. Advocates of euthanasia want self-determination, but unwittingly also foster paternalism.

Everyone who lives in the Netherlands should ask the question: why we do not return to the law? What is wrong with abiding by the Dutch euthanasia law from now on? Termination of life on request is

---

[167] Hub Zwart, *Weg met de ethiek? Filosofische beschouwingen over geneeskunde en ethiek*, Amsterdam, Thesis Publishers, 1995, p. 125-126 [Out with ethics? Philosophical observations on medicine and ethics.

permitted, termination of life without request is not.

This means we exercise more restraint when we judge other people's lives than when we judge our own. This requires that we resign ourselves to the fact a person may have to continue to live in a situation in which we would perhaps ask for euthanasia, or at least from our current situation think we would ask for euthanasia. This compels us to accept that a person lives on as long as he lives on, even if we don't know what the point of this life is.

This is where equanimity helps. Equanimity is a useful attitude when the suffering of someone close to you turns your life into an emotional rollercoaster.

Equanimity means: you do not have to fix what you cannot fix. We are not always required to act.